DRUG GAMES

Terry and Jan Todd Series on Physical Culture and Sports

Drug Games

THE INTERNATIONAL OLYMPIC COMMITTEE AND THE POLITICS OF DOPING, 1960–2008

Thomas M. Hunt

Foreword by John Hoberman

UNIVERSITY OF TEXAS PRESS
Austin

Portions of this work have been published in a different form in the following journals: *Olympika: The International Journal of Olympic Studies* and *Iron Game History: The Journal of Physical Culture.*

Requests for permission to reproduce material from this work should be sent to:

> Permissions
> University of Texas Press
> P.O. Box 7819
> Austin, TX 78713-7819
> www.utexas.edu/utpress/about/bpermission.html

✣ The paper used in this book meets the minimum requirements of ANSI/NISO Z39.48-1992 (R1997) (Permanence of Paper).

LIBRARY OF CONGRESS CATALOGING-IN-PUBLICATION DATA
Hunt, Thomas M.
    Drug games : the International Olympic Committee and the politics of doping, 1960–2008 / Thomas M. Hunt.
        p.   cm.
    Includes bibliographical references and index.
    ISBN 978-0-292-73749-5
    1. Doping in sports.   2. International Olympic Committee.
I. Title.
    RC1230.H86   2010
    362.29—dc22

                                                        2010024164

This work is dedicated to my family.

CONTENTS

John Hoberman

FOREWORD

Given the sheer scope of the doping epidemic that has engulfed Olympic sport since the 1960s, it is tempting to ask whether the founder of the modern Olympic Games, the Baron Pierre de Coubertin, might have anticipated that widespread drug use would eventually infiltrate the world of high-performance sport. This may seem like a far-fetched speculation; most people, after all, regard doping as a recent development and do not associate the nascent sports world of the 1890s with the use of performance-enhancing drugs. This view is, however, mistaken; it was well known at the time that the long-distance cyclists of the 1890s were using dangerous drugs like heroin and strychnine. The difference between then and now is that this early doping was not regarded as an illicit practice; it was rather seen as an antidote to the extreme fatigue experienced by the elite athletes of that era.

De Coubertin's creation of the modern Olympics thus coincided with the early phase of sports medicine that included informal testing of less toxic substances such as milk, tea, and alcoholic beverages. While it is conceivable that de Coubertin could have read about such experimentation in the 1894 volume of the *Archives de physiologie normale et pathologique,* there is no evidence that he did. De Coubertin did, however, anticipate the consequences of the Olympic motto *citius, altius, fortius* ("faster, higher, stronger"), and he did so without the trepidations of today's anti-doping activists. De Coubertin knew that the modern sport for which he had created an international stage possessed an element of what he called "excess." "We know," he said in 1901, "that [sport] tends inevitably toward excess, and that this is its essence, its indelible mark." Nor was de Coubertin the only Olympic visionary in this respect. "Not to develop the latent possibilities of the human body," a famous Olympian wrote in 1919, "is a crime, since it certainly violates the law of nature." The author of this Promethean declaration was none other than Avery Brundage, president of the International Olympic Committee (IOC) from 1952 to 1972. As Thomas M. Hunt documents in this book, Brundage, unlike de Coubertin, eventually had no choice but to respond to the doping issue. As Prof. Hunt demonstrates, this response was ineffectual. With prescient fatalism, Brundage feared that directing public attention to doping techniques might "give ideas to . . . unscrupulous" athletes. It was left to Pope Pius XII to warn against the use of "gravely noxious substances" in the February 1956 issue of the IOC *Bulletin*.

Drug Games is the first and only major study of how the IOC has dealt with the doping problem as it has evolved since the 1950s. Indeed, the history of the IOC is especially important in this regard, in that its failure to address the doping crisis during the presidency of Juan Antonio Samaranch (1980–2001) contributed to the creation of the World Anti-Doping Agency (WADA), which went into operation in January 2000. WADA was the result of a negotiation between the IOC and national governments, including the United States, making the IOC a major stakeholder in a global anti-doping campaign that faces daunting obstacles to its goal of driving doping practices out of the Olympic Games and other international competitions. WADA's current engagement with the prospect of genetically manipulated athletes is one of many troubling signs that the current campaign against doping practices may well prove to be futile. Here, as elsewhere, Prof. Hunt offers careful and well-documented assessments of an Olympic sports culture that finds itself embedded in a modern world where performance enhancers of various kinds have triumphed over traditional ideas about the importance of self-restraint.

This triumph of the Performance Principle, as suggested above, can be derived from the Olympic ethos that mandates the linear progress of human athletic performances for as long as such performances are possible. De Coubertin himself intuited the appeal of this dynamic principle and pointedly scorned the "anti-sporting utopians" who had intuited its dangers. The modern descendants of these "utopians" are those members of WADA who actually believe they can restrain the use of doping practices in a meaningful way and who oppose any techniques they deem to be "contrary to the spirit of sport." This is a difficult position that confronts the illicit drug use of many, many elite athletes, including many Olympians, in recent years. In February 2010, frustrations resulting from this conflict between temptation and ethical rigor led the longtime WADA-president Richard Pound to denounce doping athletes as "sociopathic cheats." At the same time, Mr. Pound and other tenacious opponents of doping must confront the possibility that de Coubertin himself defined and determined "the spirit of sport" long before it ever occurred to the IOC that it now confronted the task of reining in the "excess" the First Olympian had declared to be good.

ACKNOWLEDGMENTS

Every historian confronts temporal, financial, and intellectual limitations. Throughout the course of this project, numerous individuals helped me overcome these challenges. I owe each of them my gratitude. The staff members of several institutions patiently led me through the wealth of documentation at their respective institutions. These included the International Olympic Committee Library and Archives in Lausanne, Switzerland; the United States Olympic Committee Library and Archives in Colorado Springs, Colorado; and the University of Texas at Austin's Dolph Briscoe Center for American History and H. J. Lutcher Stark Center for Physical Culture and Sport. The IOCLA also provided access to microfilm copies of the Avery Brundage Collection, the actual documents of which are held at the University of Illinois at Urbana-Champaign. Finally, the Foundation Board of the World Anti-Doping Agency provided an enormous gift to researchers when it decided to publish online the meeting minutes of the new agency.

At the University of Texas Press, Allison Faust, Sarah Hudgens, and Lynne Chapman patiently and skillfully guided this project through the publication process. Thanks as well to Lindsay Starr and Nancy Bryan. Sue Carter performed an editorial miracle in the final stages of this project; I will never forget her diligence and patience. Mark Dyreson, Maureen Smith, and an anonymous reviewer provided an enormous service in their thoughtful critiques of an earlier version of this manuscript. Mark and his wife JoDee also deserve special thanks for showing me on multiple occasions that parenthood does not necessarily prohibit scholarship.

I also benefited from an extraordinarily supportive group of colleagues and friends at the University of Texas at Austin. My understanding of the complicated structure of Olympic governance benefited greatly from the thoughts of Professor Carla Costa. Professor H. W. Brands took time away from his own work to offer unique insights into the writing process. Professor John Hoberman met with me on numerous occasions to discuss the inner workings of international sport and generously provided me access to his own extensive research collection on performance enhancement in society. Kim Beckwith, Cindy Slater, Scott Jedlicka, Matt Bowers, Peter Ullman, Andy Miller, Stacy Metzler, and Geoff Schmalz provided much-appreciated support during the course of this project. Outside the university, Anthony Daywood, Eric Perlmutter, and Desiree Harguess gave friendship and advice on countless occasions.

Words cannot express my gratitude to Professors Jan and Terry Todd. Throughout our time together, they helped me to fashion my diverse interests in history, law, and sport policy into a workable research program. Far exceeding what could reasonably be expected of a mentor, Professor Jan Todd deserves special thanks for carefully and consistently leading me through the challenges involved in the writing of this book.

My mother and father, Laurie and Thomas L. Hunt, have spent the last thirty-two years encouraging my intellectual and personal development; my accomplishments reflect their dedication. A promising scholar in his own right, my brother Jonathan offered his own views whenever I needed a fresh perspective. Finally, my wife Hilary provided unfailing support throughout my research and writing even though it meant putting many of her dreams temporarily on hold.

DRUG GAMES

INTRODUCTION

U ntil recently, diplomatic historians have demonstrated little enthusiasm for sophisticated, archive-based studies of sport and international relations.[1] Moreover, political scientists have refrained almost entirely from integrating athletics into their theories about the nature of the international political system.[2] Members of the microfield of sport history have with few exceptions isolated themselves from both groups.[3] Former National Security Council member Victor D. Cha lamented, "If the operative question is how sport 'fits' into our understanding of world politics, then the bottom line is that the existing literature offers no clear or consistent answers."[4]

Reflecting this general underdevelopment, the few works of scholarly note on performance enhancement in sport have generally been limited in their temporal coverage, attention to political processes, and employment of archival evidence.[5] Even so, the absence in the existing historiography of a comprehensive, archival source–based history on the evolution of Olympic doping policy seemed remarkable.[6] After all, the International Olympic Committee instituted the first major anti-doping program in competitive athletics, exerting a profound impact on the world's leading sports organizations.

With these considerations in mind, I initiated a research strategy that took me to documentary collections in both the United States and Switzerland. As I worked through the records held by these institutions, my interest in global politics led me away from questions pertaining to the philosophical nature of performance enhancement in athletics—currently a leading interpretive paradigm through which scholars discuss the subject.[7] This work instead attempts to connect the history of Olympic doping policy to larger global developments.

Human actors play a significant role in history, of course. Every attempt is nevertheless made to link individuals to political forces originating both within and outside the Olympic governance structure. Greatly reducing the difficulty of this analytical endeavor, the persons involved were often themselves quite conscious of these connections. In a noteworthy manifestation of this awareness, Olympic administrators throughout the period under examination repeatedly expressed the belief that they were charged to lead a sporting movement operating virtuously above an unforgiving landscape of international politics. Ultimately, this principle of regulatory independence became partially realized.

Though still subjected to the influences of nation-states, Olympic administrators developed their own administrative structures, legislative codes, and enforcement procedures. Astonishingly, national governments for the most part recognized this autonomous governance system as legitimate. From 1960 until the late 1980s, private Olympic administrators maintained substantial authority over the anti-doping policies employed at their competitions.[8]

In doing so, these officials arrogated a number of powers historically wielded only by governmental authorities. Just as national legislatures throughout the world enacted drug legislation for their respective citizens, so the IOC began in the mid-1960s to promulgate its own list of prohibited substances. At the enforcement level, Olympic officials mirrored procedures employed by law enforcement officers, conducting scientific analyses of body fluid specimens collected from potential wrongdoers. With few exceptions, governmental bodies conceded that doping disputes fell outside their legal jurisdictions; athletes competing at an Olympic competition thus carried only limited rights to public judicial review.

From the perspective of the global political system, these developments at first glance appeared to represent an erosion of state power in an area traditionally dominated by states. Such an interpretation, however, fails to appreciate the profound policy influence exerted by state governmental units. As continued to be the case in nearly every aspect of global affairs, nation-states time and again proved to be the primary actors affecting the evolution of Olympic doping policy.[9]

Engaged during the Cold War in a struggle to win the hearts and minds of the world, the United States and the Soviet Union came to view elite international athletics as part of a larger scientific rivalry. National participation in international competition offered a way to instill in their respective citizens a sense of patriotism—a task deemed requisite to success in the conflict.[10] Moreover, both superpowers conceptualized power in sport as a means of impressing allies in their respective spheres of influence. Leaders in Moscow remained especially sensitive to the possibility that sport offered the satellite nations of Eastern Europe a potential means of undermining Soviet prestige both within and outside the Eastern bloc.[11]

The idea that Olympic success was indicative of national power motivated nations on both sides of the Iron Curtain to allow regulatory jurisdiction over performance enhancement to remain in the hands of private sports authorities. Far from wishing to restrict doping in international sport, Soviet-bloc officials often actively sponsored the employment of performance-enhancing substances. Though political leaders in the United States refrained from such direct involvement, they worried over the seemingly dominant Eastern-bloc sports teams. Finding themselves in a sort of "prisoner's dilemma," they exerted little pressure on national sport organizations to confront the issue.[12] The net result was that actions taken by Olympic officials were less likely to produce tangible progress.

At first, state units played little role in the design and implementation of Olympic doping policies. After classifying doping as a major policy issue in 1960, Olympic officials found themselves negatively affected by four interrelated problems: (1) indifference to the subject among some of their colleagues, (2) scientific difficulties pertaining to the detection of certain chemicals in the human body, (3) ethical and scientific ambiguity as to the definition of "doping," and (4) political difficulties resulting from the fragmented nature of the international sport system.

International sports leaders govern through a diffuse network of independent organizations, all of which possess different interests, jurisdictions, and powers. It is easy to mistake Olympic officials as working within a hierarchical structure featuring the IOC at its apex; their governance activities actually occur through a confederation of competing institutions. Until recently, administrators at all levels of this organizational system tended to formulate doping policies with the idea of minimizing public controversy. Meaningful reforms were deferred while a series of scandals continued to plague the Olympic movement.

At one time or another, members of nearly every organization in the international sports network were rumored to have participated in doping cover-ups. As a result, the use of potentially dangerous ergogenic aids continued to spread while the IOC focused on addressing such comparatively innocuous practices as training at high altitude.[13] By the end of the 1960s, the failures in Olympic doping policy had given rise to an environment in which, as stated by *Sports Illustrated* journalist Bil Gilbert, "The doctor and the chemist [would] soon be as important to an athlete as a coach."[14]

During the 1970s, nationalism accelerated as a causal factor in the proliferation of performance-enhancing drugs among Olympic competitors. The

German Democratic Republic's infamous Stasi secret police organization, for example, instituted a state-sponsored doping regime that administered dangerous pharmacological agents to some 10,000 athletes. Notwithstanding the adoption of several progressive steps during the decade—including the institution of anabolic steroid testing at the 1976 Montreal Summer Games—Olympic officials were unable to neutralize this type of state involvement. Thus, efforts at reform within the elite sports establishment remained relatively ineffective. Compared to the resources held by national governmental units, those available to Olympic policymakers simply remained too limited to produce meaningful reform.

The influence exerted by the international political system in aligning states against anti-doping efforts gave way during the concluding stages of the Cold War. Measured throughout the course of the superpower conflict principally in terms of raw geopolitical power, status in the emerging world order now derived to a greater extent from one's reputation for fairness and responsibility. National authorities began to take an increasingly direct role in combating performance-enhancing substances in international sport.[15]

Governmental authorities usually enact major policy changes only after the occurrence of what political scientists call a "focusing event."[16] Catalyzing the fervor for doping reform on the part of national units, such a focusing event occurred when Canadian sprinter Ben Johnson failed a test for anabolic steroids after setting a new world record in the 100-meter sprint at the 1988 Seoul Olympic Games. In light of a subsequent investigation of the episode by the Canadian national government, Olympic leaders worried that their movement might be subjected to unwanted political intrusions unless meaningful steps were taken to address the problem of doping. In response to the tangible threat that governmental units might take complete regulatory control over the issue, momentum finally built over the course of the next decade for the creation of a quasi-independent agency to oversee international doping policy.[17]

With its funding and management split between national political units and the global sporting community, the World Anti-Doping Agency went into operation in November 1999 under a mandate to implement a universal drug regulation strategy.[18] In order to maintain its autonomy from the IOC and the other components of the Olympic community, the new agency underwent a difficult process of consolidating power over performance enhancement in international sport for most of the next decade. The partnership between national political units and private sports organizations in this regulatory framework represented a critical shift in the politics of doping. Thus, systemic changes in world affairs led to a more unified policy environment for anti-doping initiatives.

The anti-doping effort of the Olympic movement developed within a dynamic, multilayered framework. International Olympic Committee leaders have varied in their commitment to anti-doping. From the beginning, the governance structure of the Olympic movement was too fragmented to allow for an effective, centralized approach to anti-doping. Complicating that governance structure has been the interface between IOC anti-doping practices and other national and international sport institutions—as well as national governments. Each of these points of interface have provided fertile ground for conflicting spheres of jurisdiction. Far above this amalgamation of competing institutional interests, global geopolitical forces have set the stage for how doping—and the athlete who participates in such practices—is to be perceived: patriot, or cheat? Finally, the array of doping substances and activities has continued to expand, forever stretching the capacity of scientists to construct means of testing. As we look to the future, toward heretofore unimagined scenarios of genetically altered athletes, the early history of doping in the Olympics offers some insights into the forces behind the progress—and stagnation—of anti-doping policy in sport.

One   DEFINING THE PROBLEM

O n August 26, 1960, twenty-three-year-old Danish cyclist Knud Jensen, riding in the 100-kilometer team time trial in that year's Rome Olympic Games, fell from his bike and fractured his skull on the pavement below. Several hours later, he died. Medical responders at first attributed the tragedy to a cerebral hemorrhage caused by heatstroke. The relatively mild temperatures that Friday and suspiciously similar collapses by two of Jensen's teammates, however, raised questions among those who followed the event. Alberto Oberholzer, director of the hospital where the cyclists received treatment, noted that it "seemed strange" that only the Danes experienced difficulty with the heat.[1]

Those more informed regarding artificial performance enhancement among competitive cyclists demonstrated no such puzzlement. In a phone call to his mother, for example, American participant Michael Hiltner described the use of stimulants by the Danish squad as common knowledge in the cycling community.[2] Olympic officials and representatives of the Danish team initially denied these rumors. However, on Sunday, August 28, Ferdinando Cocucci, Rome's deputy attorney general, announced the launch of an investigation and declared that the "authorities did not exclude the possibility" that the team had used performance-enhancing substances.[3] On the same day, a Danish newspaper reported that Oluf Jorgensen, trainer of the Danish Olympic cycling team, had admitted providing the athletes with Roniacol, a peripheral vasodilator known to enhance blood circulation.[4] Media reports about Jensen's autopsy later asserted the presence of the substance along with an assortment of amphetamines documented to stimulate cardiac output and central nervous system drive.[5] Regulatory measures implemented in response to the tragedy were weakened by a "pass-the-buck" mentality among most policymakers involved in elite athletics. Officials at the IOC, which sat at the pinnacle of the international sport governance structure, approached doping either as a public relations problem or, worse still, as someone else's responsibility. In addition, they resisted centralized responsibility for doping policy creation and execution by the IOC, rationalizing this avoidance by the stated objective of protecting the IOC from the organizational, financial, and legal consequences of such a role.

The international federations, national Olympic committees, and organizing committees for Olympic competitions, thus endowed with the responsibility to develop doping controls, were either indifferent to or actually encouraged the use of drugs. Within the United States and among its Communist rivals, a "sportive nationalism" blinded sport officials to the urgency of the problem.[6] Indeed, a transfer of America's "containment doctrine" to the private realm of international athletics—including the Olympics—provided an impetus to American athletes and sports officials to adopt pharmacological techniques employed by Eastern-bloc teams. In addition, U.S. governmental officials did not push the nation's private sports organizations to reform; sporting success loomed larger in their minds than the elimination of doping.

Although IOC president Avery Brundage protested after Knud Jensen's death that "I've been connected with sports for sixty years, and I'd never considered such a thing," Brundage had, in fact, been aware of the increasing use of performance-enhancing substances in elite athletics for a considerable period prior to the cyclist's collapse.[7] A 1951 issue of the IOC's regularly published *Bulletin du Comité International Olympique,* for example, included a response by the International Rowing Federation to accusations that the Danish rowing team had used "poison" to win the 1950 European Championships. Protesting that it possessed no jurisdiction over the issue, the federation went on to claim that the Association of Danish Doctors was responsible for determining whether the squad's use of "a daily dose of three tablets of Anrostin [*sic*] during twelve days can be considered as 'doping.'"[8] Brundage and other Olympic policymakers by then also knew of a decision—as demonstrated by its publication in the *Bulletin* in 1951—by the International Boxing Federation to prohibit the administration "immediately before or during a contest of drugs or chemical substances not forming part of the normal diet of a boxer."[9]

Rather than taking preventive action in light of these developments, the IOC did nothing, and at the 1952 Winter Olympic Games, several speed skaters became ill due to their excessive use of amphetamine stimulants.[10] In addition, the surprisingly successful Soviet weightlifting team at that year's Summer Games in Helsinki—the first in which the Soviets competed—prompted the dismayed American coach Bob Hoffman to publicly

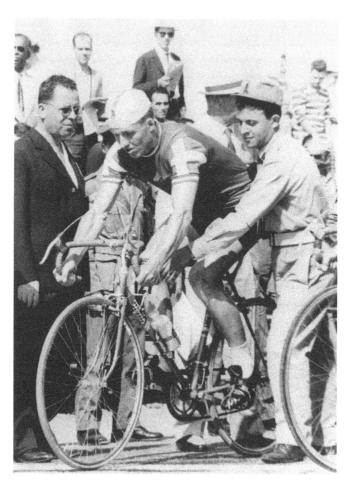

FIGURE I.   *Danish cyclist Knud Enemark Jensen (1936–1960) before the start of the 100-kilometer team trial at the Rome Olympics, August 26, 1960 (Keystone/Hulton Archive/Getty Images).*

accuse its members of artificial enhancement. "I know they're taking that hormone stuff to increase their strength," he said.[11]

Hoffman's suspicions were validated in a Viennese tavern at the 1954 World Weightlifting Championships. During a break in the competition, a Soviet team physician "after a few drinks" informed his American counterpart John Ziegler that "some members of his team were using testosterone" to add muscle mass. The effects were so dramatic that Ziegler believed the Soviets must be "abusing the drugs [so] heavily" that they were "having to get catheterized."[12] The episode intrigued Ziegler, who began to experiment with synthetic testosterone upon his return to the United States. He took the substance himself and gave it to a small number of weightlifters in order to test its performance-enhancing effects. Although Ziegler soon abandoned his use of testosterone, his hopes for a new pharmacological agent were soon realized. In 1958, the CIBA pharmaceutical company announced the production of a new synthetic anabolic steroid, developed to help burn victims and geriatric patients.[13] Given the trade name Dianabol, it possessed fewer androgenic side effects than testosterone but retained the desired anabolic benefits. Soon thereafter, Ziegler convinced three high-ranking U.S. weightlifters to begin using Dianabol, and all three experienced significant improvements in both strength and muscle mass. Following this success, the use of Dianabol spread rapidly among U.S. lifters and, from there, to other sports.[14]

Given the Cold War impetus for the United States to keep pace with its Communist rivals in the Olympic medals race, a few American athletes very likely joined in the use of ergogenic substances earlier than 1958. At the 1956 Summer Games in Melbourne, for example, it was rumored among some of the competitors that several members of the United States track-and-field squad were using testosterone.[15] Despite these reports, however, the various organizations that constituted the Olympic governance structure refused to take definitive steps in the 1950s to impede the proliferation of doping. This held true regardless of the nation in which an actual or alleged drug scandal occurred. When an American physician mentioned amphetamines during a discussion of British runner Roger Bannister's sub-four-minute mile, sports officials immediately rejected the possibility; an actual investigation was preposterous.[16]

Yet, the topic of doping began to attract the attention of prominent figures outside the sports world. Pope Pius XII, for instance, wrote in the February 1956 issue of the IOC *Bulletin* that "one must deplore the error . . . of absorb[ing] gravely noxious substances. Such is the case when consuming highly stimulating drugs which . . . are looked upon as a kind of fraud by specialists." Criticizing the tacit acceptance of ergogenic aids among the members of the Olympic community, the Pope concluded that "the responsibility of spectators, organisers and the press is very serious when they encourage this risky practice."[17]

Brundage received a further warning from Harvard medical professor Henry K. Beecher at a 1959 American Medical Association conference in Dallas, Texas. After the meeting, Beecher sent him several articles on the use of amphetamines by competitive athletes. Brundage, whose attention to ethical matters centered on questions of amateurism rather than biomedical debates, responded by outlining the complexity of the international sports system, which made any strategy for dealing with performance-enhancing drugs virtually impossible. "When you inquire how we are going to solve this problem," Brundage wrote in early 1960, "you pose a most difficult question. The initial responsibility is in the hands of the National Federations of a score or more sports in more than ninety countries . . . [among whom] there may be some who are unscrupulous." Aggressive action, he continued, might only exacerbate the situation in that "if we inaugurate a campaign of education it may give ideas to the unscrupulous ones referred to above."[18] Believing that pharmacological doping was of relatively minor importance, Brundage and his colleagues on the IOC saw little reason to expend the monetary and managerial resources to overcome these obstacles.

By early 1960, the problem of exogenous performance enhancement had become so acute that President Brundage felt it necessary to address the issue in an IOC meeting in San Francisco. He related the disturbing "use in certain sport circles" of a pharmacological agent called "Amphetamine Sulfate," which, he continued, "is nothing else but a dope or a drug."[19] IOC delegate Bo Eklund suggested a rigorous scientific investigation of the issue. However, the committee ignored the recommendation in favor of a more modest proposal: the members of the committee, few of whom had any medical training, should "speak of this matter in their respective countries." No further actions were specified.[20]

In retrospect, the IOC's passivity on the issue prior to the tragedy in Rome seems irresponsible. However, it should be remembered that doping had long been an accepted practice in competitive athletics. Until the Cold War, ergogenic aids were for the most part accepted as tools through which to expand physical and cognitive abilities.[21] In fact, the first known instance of doping in the modern Olympics occurred fifty-six years prior to Jensen's death, when Thomas Hicks, an American runner, ingested a mixture of strychnine, brandy, and raw eggs before the marathon at the 1904 Games in St. Louis. Hicks's performance so impressed U.S. sports authority Charles Lucas that he declared, "The Marathon race, from a medical standpoint, demonstrated that drugs are of much benefit to athletes."[22]

Even then, however, the dangers of doping were apparent. Lucas described Hicks's collapse at the finish line: "His eyes were dull, lusterless, the ashen color of his face and skin had deepened; his arms appeared as weights well tied down; he could scarcely lift his legs, while his knees were almost stiff."[23] Lucas believed these risks were worth taking, however, contending that American athletes should be lauded for endangering their bodies by employing ergogenic aids in service to the nation. Lucas expressed this principle in condemning a fellow competitor who crossed the finish line ahead of Hicks after riding part of the course in the passenger seat of an automobile. That reprehensible individual, Lucas declared, "robbed a man who, four miles out on the road, was running the last ounces of strength out of his body, kept in mechanical action by the use of drugs, that he might bring America the Marathon honors."[24] The runner who rode in an automobile was just a cheat. Hicks, by contrast, put his own health at risk for his country. Lucas's characterization of drug use by athletes as a sign of patriotism can be seen in succeeding generations of national leaders.

Jensen's death, however, finally forced Olympic leaders to engage with the problem on a meaningful level. In the aftermath of the tragedy in Rome, the IOC executive board became more attentive to the danger posed by unregulated doping. Meeting in Rome fifteen days after Jensen's collapse, members of the group asserted that the Olympic movement "deplores deeply the death of a Danish cyclist competing in the present Games." Perhaps more importantly, they worried that the fatality might damage the prestige of the Olympic movement. Brundage felt particularly displeased by the public relations debacle that ensued after Jensen was posthumously awarded a gold medal.[25] The board, struggling to correct the impression that an Olympic athlete had been honored for doping, called for the implementation of punitive measures (to be carried out by some other, undefined organization). "The responsible parties ought to be penalized," the board declared. As for the IOC, the board simply asked Danish sports officials for a report on the situation so that a definitive decision could be made sometime in the future.[26] Beyond this tepid response to the public relations disaster occasioned by Jensen's death, very little was done to address the growing problem of doping.

This lack of substantive action would become a familiar pattern in the IOC's approach to the issue over the next several decades. The activities of IOC officials were to a large degree restricted to attempts to define the ethical and scientific boundaries of the problem. Among these, initiatives to create a universal policy approach for its solution remained entirely absent.

Over a year later, convening in Athens in June of 1961, the IOC executive board finally revisited the problem when French delegate Comte Jean de Beaumont argued that the Olympic movement needed some form of policy toward performance-enhancing drugs so that future deaths could be prevented. The board accordingly agreed to submit to the upcoming IOC general session the question of whether a doping control system should be established.[27] In that meeting, President Brundage again referred to the seriousness of the situation and asserted that "sanctions should be applied." However, in a statement that reflected the ethical and scientific uncertainty of Olympic policymakers on the issue, he argued that the IOC should first decide exactly what "constitutes a doping."[28] In January 1962, believing that he needed help from medical experts to resolve confusion over the definition, he wrote to IOC chancellor Otto Mayer that "the problem of 'doping' is not a simple one and we must have professional advice on where to draw the line. This is a difficult problem. I shall appoint a subcommittee of doctors . . . to deal with the subject."[29]

Brundage's decision to seek help from the scientific community was prudent. A graduate of the University of Illinois and the founder of a successful construction company in Chicago, he possessed extensive experience in Olympic governance; however, he lacked the medical training requisite to a knowledgeable stance on doping issues. As for his moral compass regarding the subject, Brundage was deeply committed to the transnational ideals of the Olympic movement. For him, the Olympic movement served as a universal religion through which international peace could be accomplished by means of athletic competition. Reflecting upon the principles ascribed to the modern Olympic movement, Brundage declared that as its founder, "Pierre de Coubertin did no more than consider sport as a universal philosophy in which all men could communicate, wherever they come from and whatever their circumstances."[30] Throughout his life, Brundage remained dedicated to this ideal. His conviction that participation in the movement advanced humankind's progress toward global harmony at times appeared naïve—most notoriously in his opposition to calls for a boycott of the 1936 "Nazi Olympics" while he was head of the American Olympic Association.[31]

Brundage's idealism was accompanied by an interpersonal style that some found severe. Remarking on his relationship with Brundage, IOC member Arthur Porritt stated, "I knew him very well, but I never got close to him. I liked him and I trusted him, but I could never call him a friend." According to fellow IOC member Herman van Karnebeek, Brundage "never visited anybody, never went to anybody's house." These characteristics created a barrier between Brundage and the other members of the IOC. "He lived in a castle of his own," Porritt asserted, "and you had to get the portcullis [up] before you could get in."[32] In times of crisis, Brundage could, in addition, be pragmatic to the point of viciousness. Prior to his assumption of the IOC presidency in 1972, for instance, he insisted that his name remain absent on the birth certificates of two male children born out

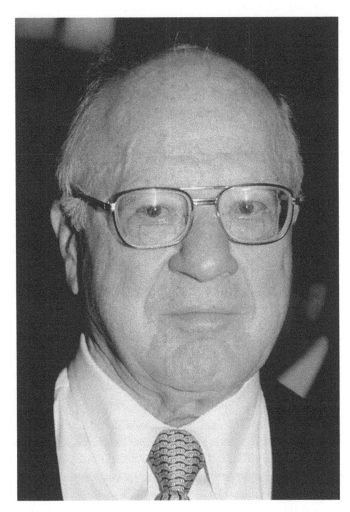

FIGURE 2.   *Avery Brundage, president of the International Olympic Committee
from 1952 to 1972, January 1, 1973 (STAFF/AFP/Getty Images).*

of wedlock. Brundage forbade the pair from ever identifying him as their
father; they were given nothing in his will.[33]

In the end, Brundage failed to appreciate the saliency of doping, giving greater priority to other organizational and political issues that he perceived as requiring more immediate attention. The issue of doping was lost
in the diffuse governance structure of the Olympic movement, and the
establishment of an effective, centralized IOC regulatory approach was
forestalled.[34]

In March 1962, the IOC agreed to create a new doping subcommittee, with Dr. Arthur Porritt, then president of the Royal College of Surgeons of England, as its head. The group, it was suggested, would coordinate its activities with the Fédération Internationale de Médecine du Sport (FIMS), a body with which the IOC had remained loosely affiliated since it was "officially recognized" by the Olympics in 1952.[35] The choice of Porritt was curious, however; at the IOC session in St. Moritz in 1948, he had argued against any involvement by the IOC with questions of a medical or scientific nature. "Any direct action in this connection," he believed, "would but lead the Committee into spheres where it is neither justified nor equipped to enter . . . As a corporate body we have neither the right nor the machinery to play any direct or practical part."[36] In addition, the subcommittee initially received little organizational support from the IOC, and Chancellor Mayer wrote to two of its members, warning that "there will be some difficulties for you to meet as you all live in different parts of the world."[37]

Porritt, in one of his few accomplishments as head of the subcommittee, responded by appointing to the group Dr. Pierre Krieg, who as a resident of the Olympic movement's home city of Lausanne, Switzerland, would be able to "keep a closer contact with the chancellery of the I.O.C."[38] Even this modest act, however, indirectly served to demonstrate Porritt's weakness. IOC chancellor Mayer had actually initiated the appointment by suggesting to the British physician that Krieg might be useful for this role. "I can assure you that he is a clever man," Mayer wrote, "and he might do a good work [sic]." "He [rather than you] could report straight to us and it would give a stronger contact between the IOC, and your commission."[39] Mayer was also dismayed by Porritt's decision to skip the IOC general session in June of 1962, writing to him, "As you are not coming to Moscow, it is of no use to call a meeting there." The chancellor's exhortations to Porritt suggest that Mayer was frustrated with both Porritt's performance and the general tendency among IOC members to see doping as a problem of image management rather than as a medical or ethical issue, as well as their habit of shifting responsibility for its management to other organizations. "Something must be done as quickly as possible so that we can show to the World . . . that the I.O.C. does something," Mayer wrote to Porritt. "It will be also a great help to the International Federations" in formulating policies for the use of performance-enhancing drugs among their athletes.[40]

Porritt's ambivalence toward doping was further demonstrated when he missed the IOC general session in Moscow; one of his colleagues on the doping subcommittee, Dr. Ferreira Santos, took his place in submitting a report to the body.[41] Porritt's subsequent inactivity did little to persuade

Olympic policymakers of his commitment. Mayer wrote angrily on September 27, 1962, "Since our Moscow Session where we have elected a special commission on Doping, of which you are President, we have not heard anything! Would you kindly let me know when you expect to send us a report from the Commission."[42] In late October—nearly a month later—Porritt meekly responded, "Here I am, at last, with many apologies . . . but I have just returned" from two extensive tours of Africa and the United States. "This is the sort of thing," he continued, "that has made it quite impossible for me to do much about the Doping Commission." Porritt noted that he would "do what I can as soon as I can, but I really have very little spare time these days." He suggested that a colleague on the commission "who seems to have shown some interest," should take his place as chair and that the IOC should "see what he can do."[43]

The IOC leadership, who had wanted a report defining doping before the 1964 Games began in Tokyo, was frustrated with Porritt's continued inaction. Brundage wrote Porritt that "inasmuch as Dr. Santos has already assembled some material and brought in a partial report I think we should ask him to head the Commission."[44] Under Santos, the doping subcommittee published a report in a 1963 issue of the IOC *Bulletin*. Doping, according to the report, could be defined as

> an illegal procedure used by certain athletes, in the form of drugs; physical means and exceptional measures which are used by small groups in a sporting community in order to alter positively or negatively the physical or physiological capacity of a living creature, man or animal in competitive sport.[45]

Of course, the inclusion of performance inhibition, as well as the vague terminology with regard to "physical means" and "exceptional measures," left substantial room for interpretation. Most importantly, the definition was not tied to a formal regulatory policy under the auspices of the IOC.

1964 TOKYO OLYMPIC GAMES

At the same time, Brundage was again arguing that the international federations that governed the various sports in the Olympic movement—and not the IOC—should hold primary responsibility for promulgating doping policies. Brundage's philosophy of dispersed regulatory authority over performance enhancement exerted powerful sway over

IOC decision making during his twenty-year term as president. Writing to Mayer, he asserted that "it would be better for us to cooperate with organizations more competent to treat on the subject of 'doping' than we are."[46] This recommendation went against those issued by both the European Council on Doping and the Biological Preparation of the Athlete Taking Part in Competitive Sports. In a January 1963 meeting in Uriage, France, this latter assembly of biologists, lawyers, sports leaders, athletes, physicians, pharmacists, and journalists developed what it felt was a "reasonable and realistic anti-doping plan of battle." Calling first for the creation of an international commission on doping, the council insisted that "it is urgent and vital that an international body should examine the matter thoroughly and standardize the rules governing sport in the different countries." The use of performance-enhancing drugs, according to the council, constituted "an infringement of rights or offence in sport," which could, despite a few contrary opinions, be successfully curtailed in that "there are efficacious means of detecting the use of artificial stimulants."[47]

Nevertheless, the IOC continued to insist upon its lack of jurisdiction and to argue that the international and national sports federations were the only organizations that could address the issue. In November of 1963, the IOC pronounced that "the main struggle is only just beginning, and it will intensify . . . by reason of the comprehension and the severity of the sporting federations."[48] Several months later, increasingly aware that this posture was doing little to help the image of the movement, IOC members again deliberated the matter in Innsbruck, Austria, at their sixty-first general session. Bo Eklund, again framing the policy problem as a public relations issue, suggested that "in order to stop Press reports about athletes doping, blood tests could be taken in suspicious cases." And, Santos having died, the doping subcommittee was once again hindered by the ineffectual leadership of Porritt, who reported at the Innsbruck meeting that "it was a little too soon to comment on the question. Probably the next year there would be great benefits forthcoming from proved medical advice."[49]

There was, not surprisingly, little policy development on the issue of ergogenic aids prior to the 1964 Tokyo Games. A limited number of chemical analyses were conducted in the cycling events at those competitions, so that Porritt and the IOC executive board could—somewhat to their own surprise—claim that "it seems that tests have been made in Tokyo."[50] American track-and-field star Harold Connolly would later testify that these tests were ineffective. In a 1973 U.S. Senate hearing, he recalled that his roommate brought his own drugs, which were "boldly presented . . . to the medical staff of the team." Reluctant to give an advantage to squads representing rival nations, the staff members "placed the drug in their refrigerator and the team nurse gave him the injections . . . Our Olympic medical staff were really not very concerned with what he was receiving."[51]

However tentative the testing efforts at the Tokyo Games may have been, they represented the first instance of concrete action taken to combat doping in the Olympic movement. Moreover, the targeting of cycling was quite perceptive in that cycling was the sport most overrun by performance-enhancing drugs in this era. The International Cycling Union and its head, Adriano Rodini, were of course displeased with the protocol, and a series of complaints were quickly fired off to Brundage.[52] The surprisingly confident president of the IOC, however, reminded the executive board of the perils of doping in terms of "the degradation of sport" and asserted that "any degrated [sic] sport would be expelled from the Games."[53]

Finally convinced that the issue deserved his full attention, Porritt exhibited greater concern about doping at the 1965 IOC general session in Tokyo. He suggested that the delegates should construct and implement four interconnected policies. The IOC should, first, issue a formal declaration denouncing the use of any performance-enhancing drug; second, create regulations that would allow "sanctions against any [National Olympic Committee] or any person who directly or indirectly promoted the use of drugs"; third, insist that those committees require their athletes to submit to "an examination at any time"; and finally, append to the application forms for Olympic participation the clause, "I do not use drugs, and hereby declare that I am prepared to submit to any examination that may be thought necessary." After further declaring his belief that a team of medical practitioners should attend future Games "to carry out very precise and very rapid examinations," Porritt suggested that "the International Federations should also be asked for their support." Here, Porritt was demonstrating a subtle but noteworthy shift from earlier IOC language, which gave sole responsibility to the federations as opposed to calling for their "support." The attendees thereafter unanimously condemned the practice of doping and called for the executive board to incorporate their decision into "a more precise text for the rules of eligibility" for participation in the Olympics.[54]

ALTITUDE TRAINING AS DOPING

During the mid-1960s, IOC members added high-altitude physiology to their existing ethical debates regarding the science of elite international athletics.[55] At a meeting of the committee in October 1963, delegates voiced questions as to the potential difficulties that athletes might face should Mexico City, a leading candidate for the 1968 Summer Olympic Games, obtain the rights to host the competitions. Constructed atop the ancient Aztec capital of Tenochtitlán, the metropolis, after all, sat nearly 7,500 feet above sea level. Attuned to the economic benefits of ever faster times, IOC leaders worried in particular over a possible repeat of the disappointing performances witnessed at the 1955 Pan-American Games in Mexico City.[56] The Mexican delegation attempted to allay concerns about decreased performances due to the difficulties related to elevation by questioning their scientific validity and by promising to reimburse athletes for expenses involved with the acclimatization process.[57] At the 1964 Tokyo meeting, General José de J. Clark Flores, chair of the Organizing Committee for the Mexico City Olympic Games, again criticized those who argued that the altitude of the Mexican capital would hurt the competitions, claiming that their worries were "just a question of prejudice." Continuing this line of reasoning, Clark reassured his audience that "no accidents had ever been recorded" among competitors performing at high altitudes and that in the unlikely event anyone actually became sick, "after a few days . . . [they would be] perfectly alright."[58]

The other contenders for the 1968 Summer Olympics—Lyon, Detroit, and Buenos Aires—likewise received a series of questions from the IOC relating to "size, population, climate, [and] altitude." Seeking to benefit from the perceived disadvantages of Mexico City's altitude, the representatives of these locations emphasized the attractiveness of their comparatively moderate elevations. Officials from Buenos Aires, for instance, stressed that all events could be conveniently held at sea level if their cities won the bid competition.[59] Taking a firm stance against this implied criticism, the Mexicans argued that the elevation of their proposed site would have a "harmless effect . . . on the athlete's cardiopulmonary capacity, even though they come from lower altitudes."[60]

When the time came for a decision as to the location of the XIXth Olympiad, General Clark repeated his assurances to IOC delegates that Mexico City's altitude would pose little problem from a physiological standpoint and that the organizing committee would be more than happy to pay whatever costs athletes might face with regard to their adjustment to high-altitude competition. Finally having persuaded an adequate number of delegates to support Mexico City's candidacy, Clark rejoiced with his colleagues after receiving official word as to the success of their bid at the 60th IOC general session in Baden-Baden, Germany; indeed, having put together a remarkable bid, the Mexican capital secured the right to host the competitions by a comfortable margin, receiving thirty out of a possible fifty-eight votes.[61]

American sport officials remained worried, however, about the potentially detrimental effects of Mexico City's location upon the performance of their athletes. Jim Swarts, a delegate of the United States Olympic Committee from the National Collegiate Athletic Association, recommended that the committee consult a physician who "is an expert on the effects of altitude on athletes."[62] Harry McPhee, a physician who according to USOC president Kenneth L. Wilson "guided us with great skill through a number of Olympiads," warned that "I don't know whether you gentlemen understand [that] the problem we will have there is one of oxygen and oxygen is the one element which the body can't store."[63] After one delegate concluded that "it seems to be mandatory that we do everything we can to in [sic] further experiments and research under conditions most closely similar to those . . . in Mexico City," a number of alternatives were discussed.[64] These included involvement with several sports medicine projects then under way; as Swarts put it, "When it comes to the research side of it in todays [sic] situation you might as well argue against motherhood and the American flag."[65] One sees in these words the linkages made by national Olympic authorities between science, sport, and national prestige.

As for the relationship of high-altitude training to doping, the USOC leadership asked one of its delegates, physician Daniel Hanley, about "any medicine available that will facilitate adaption [sic]" to altitude. Responding that "there is one that may, as a matter of fact," Hanley cautioned that "this part of the adaptation would be this much [a small part] in the total scheme . . . and we have not [yet] translated the use of these drugs into the human blood."[66] In addition, IOC officials, who were increasingly wary of the chemical and scientific steps being proposed to accommodate the Mexico City location, devised a policy that would restrict such efforts. At an IOC meeting in Rome, Lord David Burghley, the Marquess of Exeter, proposed a rule stating that "in order to achieve fairness as far as possible between competitors, no athletes other than those who normally live at such heights, shall train specially at high altitudes more than 6 weeks up to the start of their event, in the last three months before the Games." Showing his idealism, Burghley continued, "To break this rule would be a gross breach of good sportsmanship and it is sure that no-one . . . would wish in any way to be guilty of taking an unfair advantage over other competitors."[67]

In light of the relationship between altitude and the physiology of performance, it was somewhat odd that the IOC leadership chose to address altitude training as an issue of amateurism rather than as a medical problem; the doping subcommittee, observing simply that "the Commission notes with interest this decision," was not involved.[68] Under the regulations in force at the time, no athlete could leave work to train for more than four weeks a year and still compete in an Olympic competition. Seeing some sense in applying this standard to the question of high-altitude preparation, IOC delegates meeting in Rome during the spring of 1966 revised Burghley's rule and announced that Olympians could train at altitude for only one month prior to the Mexico City Games.[69] The new USOC president, Douglas Roby, noted that the new regulation would affect the strategies employed by his organization. The rule, he stated, "moulds or somewhat shapes our thinking as to what we are going to do in preparation for the Mexico City Games."[70] Still, he said later, "I don't think there is going to be any policing on this . . . I don't think anybody will be penalized."[71]

In the larger context of the Cold War, Western countries were becoming increasingly suspicious that Communist-bloc scientists were seeking the type of physiological edge that the Marquess of Exeter was trying to combat. In April of 1967, the London *Observer* reported that despite official pronouncements to the contrary by Konstantin Andranov, president of the USSR's national Olympic committee, the Soviets were operating a high-altitude training facility deep within the Tien Shan Mountains in western Kyrgyzstan. Directed by Leningrad's Central Institute of Physical Culture, psychologists, physiologists, and, most ominously, pharmacologists were working to determine an optimal system of high-altitude preparation. Performance-enhancing drugs, it seems, were a central part of this operation. As revealed by Felix Talyshev, secretary of the institute, "We must," in addition to normal athletic training, "also pay attention to pharmacological preparations." The *Observer* cited a Russian newspaper as stating that "there lies a grain of truth in the saying that Mexico will be the scientists' and not the athletes' Olympic Games." The Soviets, the *Observer* article concluded, "might be experimenting with various forms of doping, either to overcome the effects of altitude, [or] to improve performance generally."[72]

In the end, and after much criticism by other members of the Olympic establishment, Brundage and Burghley relented and allowed an extra two weeks of training. Again conflating the subjects of amateurism and altitude physiology, a final—though complicated—decision was released by the IOC in August of 1967. The regulation first stated that "we want to make it plain that, although it is not prohibited, the general operation of special training camps is not in accordance with the spirit of amateur sport." The regulation went on to elaborate upon the committee's reasoning.

As there has been so much misinformation circulated on the effect on performance of high altitude such as that of Mexico City we have decided to make a special allowance for the year 1968 only of two weeks . . . In our eligibility code, it is provided that participation for special training in a camp for more than four weeks in any one calendar year is not permitted . . . Six weeks in special training camps during the year 1968 will be permitted but no more than four of these weeks shall be during the three months preceding the opening of the Games in October 1968.[73]

THE DOPING CRISIS CONTINUES

The USOC's response to high-altitude training revealed the deeper problem of doping among its athletes. One of the physicians in attendance at the American high-altitude training camp at South Lake Tahoe, H. Kay Dooley, openly supported the use of performance-enhancing drugs by athletes. "I don't think it is possible for a weight man to compete internationally without using anabolic steroids," he argued. Although he denied prescribing steroids at the camp, Dooley acknowledged that "I also did not inquire what the boys were doing on their own. I did not want to be forced into a position of having to report them for use of a banned drug. A physician involved in sports must keep the respect and confidence of the athletes with whom he is working." As for any moral dilemma posed by the adoption of such a position, Dooley remained unmoved. "I see no reason not to make it available to an athlete," he asserted. "I can't see any ethical difference between giving a drug to improve performance and wrapping an ankle or handing out a salt pill for the same purpose."[74] Tom Waddell, a decathlete who trained at the camp, later estimated that a full third of the American track-and-field squad was using anabolic steroids.[75]

Dooley's attitude was fairly representative of the time. The mass production of pharmaceutical products meant that Americans were much more likely than their parents or grandparents had been to turn to prescription drugs for the amelioration of a variety of ills that would have gone untreated in earlier decades. Indeed, more than thirty types of pharmacological agents could be found in the average American home during the 1960s.[76] Another contributing factor to both Dooley's sanguine attitude to doping and the IOC's lack of concern was the growth of recreational drug use among young people throughout the Western world—including Olympic athletes. Marijuana, hallucinogens, and, of course, amphetamines were widely available in youth circles, leading millions of young people to experiment with various drugs associated with the counterculture.[77] By the late 1960s, recreational drug use was as much a part of the world of elite sport as it was part of the average American community.[78]

In addition, American political leaders loudly complained about the weakness of American teams in comparison to those from the Soviet Union. In the lead-up to the Tokyo Games, Senator Hubert Humphrey requested a comprehensive report from the Department of State as to the condition of Soviet athletics.[79] He proclaimed that "the Russians are feverishly building toward what they expect to be a major Cold War victory in 1964: a massive triumph in the Tokyo Olympics." Stressing the urgency of the matter, he continued, "Once they have crushed us in the coming Olympic battle, the Red propaganda drums will thunder out in a worldwide tattoo, heralding the 'new Soviet men and women' as 'virile, unbeatable conquerors' in sports—or anything else."[80] Given the pressure to win—whatever the cost—U.S. sports officials, coaches, and athletes found performance-enhancing substances to be ever more attractive.

The resulting incorporation of performance-enhancing drugs in the training regimens of elite athletes produced a policy dilemma for the IOC leadership. While meeting in Lausanne in July of 1965, the IOC executive board was informed that "a medical check [at the 1964 Tokyo Games] has proved that certain athletes had been given shots and that some teams had drugs and artificial stimulants with them." Several policies were proposed. "We ought to have a rule obliging the athletes to submit to a medical examination," the committee concluded. As for the implementation of specific punitive measures, the board declared that "if drugs and artificial stimulants have been used, the athlete or the team should be disqualified."[81] Later that year, President Brundage, who was concerned about the interpretation of such a rule, argued that the board would need to "study the question to know if the whole team must be disqualified when one of its members is convicted of using drugs . . . if this question ought to figure in our Rules and if sanctions ought to be considered."[82]

Departing slightly from his prior statements, Brundage also announced to the international federations that the IOC "would take our [own] precautions against the use of drugs . . . and penalize those who are guilty of their use."[83] In April 1966, Porritt and the doping subcommittee presented a report that included a preliminary list of substances that would be prohibited at the Mexico City Games, noting that the "problem of doping can be met only by a long-term education policy stressing the physical and moral aspects of the subject." The report recommended a series of stop-gap measures. First, the national Olympic committees should "stimulate general education on the subject" and incorporate a promise to refrain from doping within their entry forms. The international federations should, in addition, write their own rules barring the use of performance-enhancing drugs. As for the IOC, it should issue a statement against doping, "be given powers to establish sanctions against either N.O.Cs [sic] or individuals adjudged to be guilty," and make arrangements for medical tests at the Games. Control of these drugs would be especially important in Mexico City "because the athletes will not be accustomed to the high altitude." Finally, it was conclusively established that the entire team "of an athlete convicted of doping will be disqualified for the sport concerned."[84]

This modestly more aggressive IOC stance against drugs was followed several months later by Porritt's announcement of his resignation from the doping subcommittee so that he could become the new governor general of New Zealand. Porritt's departure, as well as attrition by death or termination of service on the part of most of the subcommittee members, presented an opportunity for a new organizational model.[85] This evolution, which would entail a shift in focus from "doping" to "medicine," would take some time, as Brundage and the balance of the IOC leadership deliberated on how best to address the situation. IOC secretary general J. W. Westerhoff wrote to Porritt in March 1967, stating that if Porritt wished to resign, "a new chairman has to be appointed for the sub-committee for doping, and I should very much appreciate your suggestion as to who should be your successor." Westerhoff expressed his preference for Prince Alexandre de Merode, "who, although being no medecin [sic], has shown much interest into the matter."[86]

In the meantime, President Brundage and the executive board were again attempting to transfer responsibility over doping control to the other organizations in the international sport system. At a board meeting in late October 1966, a "full discussion" over a possible Medical Congress at the 1968 Games revealed that "many of the athletes would not be prepared to undergo medical tests" at the competitions. Not wishing to bear the full brunt of the public outcry that was sure to attend the number of positive results should a comprehensive IOC testing protocol be implemented, the issue, in the executive board's estimation, should be "left to the Organizing Committee to decide."[87] Shortly after the meeting, Porritt, who remained an advisor, wrote to Brundage, "As we recognize the Fédération Internationale [de Médecine du Sport] as our official medical body, it would seem that the responsibility of arranging for possible tests during the Games should be put in their hands."[88] Nevertheless, a drug memorandum distributed to the executive board by Prince de Merode, then a member of the doping subcommittee, led to the decision that mandatory testing should be put on the agenda of the upcoming May 1967 IOC general session in Tehran.[89]

At the Tehran meeting, it was conclusively decided that Prince de Merode would take Porritt's place as chair of the new medical commission.[90] As a Belgian aristocrat, de Merode embodied the notion that the Olympic leadership should remain the preserve of the well-bred and financially secure social elite. Exuding an element of fatherly responsibility for Olympic competitors, he shied away from punitive measures that he felt were overly harsh. "Cheating will go until the end of the world," he later asserted, "but our job must be as much to expose the health dangers of depression, of glandular and cardiovascular damage, as to *ban* people."[91] Under his guidance, the IOC medical commission would do its best to limit the imposition of suspensions whenever possible.[92]

At the Tehran meeting, a list of the drugs for which there would be testing was also finalized; it included alcohol, cocaine, vasodilators, opiates, amphetamines, ephedrine, and cannabis. Although anabolic steroids were specifically referenced as constituting "'doping' from the Olympic viewpoint," they were excluded from the list, even though a report on their properties, including their known side effects, was appended to the minutes of the session. This report specified that anabolic steroids could cause jaundice, increased blood pressure, impotence, reduced sperm counts, menstrual problems, and hirsutism; they could also stunt adolescent bone growth. Anabolic steroids were excluded from the list for the simple reason that a test did not yet exist.[93]

With the 1968 Games approaching, the IOC leadership began to press the other groups in the international sports system to exhibit greater attention to the issue of performance enhancement. On August, 31, 1967, for instance, IOC secretary general J. W. Westerhoff wrote to Dr. Eduardo Hay, director general of Mexico City's Olympic sports center: "Recently, specially in connection with doping affaires [*sic*] during European and World Championships here, many disastrous things have happened, even death, and I do think we have to . . . [be] quite diligent in this matter."[94] Within the IOC itself, the transfer of authority from the doping subcommittee to the new medical commission was concluded in late September 1967. The new group, which had an expanded area of jurisdiction, met for the first time on the 25th and 26th of that month in Lausanne to consider new ways to handle the problem.[95]

The results of that meeting, however, were far from dramatic. The medical commission recommended many of the same steps that its predecessor had been advocating for the last several years: revision of the athletes' entry forms to include a promise to submit to medical examination, random drug tests, and close consultations with the international federations over the allowable time lapse between events and specimen deposits. In its sole original contribution, the medical commission did, it should be noted, take "great care to lay down a procedure for these tests," including a protocol that detailed "point by point all the various stages which must be followed from the moment a sample is taken to the moment that a laboratory has carried out its analysis."[96]

The specification of a protocol reflected several points of concern within the medical commission. First, de Merode seemed to genuinely care for the protection of athletes' rights; only a standardized set of testing and enforcement measures would satisfactorily address this sensitivity. Second, the implementation of these processes would lessen the threat of expensive and embarrassing public legal proceedings initiated by competitors in the aftermath of a failed drug analysis. The success of the testing procedures nevertheless depended largely on the actual distribution of regulatory power in the Olympic organizational framework. If administrative authority remained divided among several units, the likelihood that officials could construct an effective, fair anti-doping framework remained dim. The odds seemed to improve considerably under consolidated administrative control.

The medical commission's plan to operate anti-doping efforts entirely within the Olympic governance structure reflected the ambivalence of national authorities regarding the subject. Soviet scientists, coaches, and athletes, competing on behalf of a political regime that employed sport to enhance its perceived position in the international balance of power, eagerly sought a pharmacological advantage. U.S. government officials, if less interested in proactively developing performance-enhancing drugs and training methods, devoted relatively little attention to curtailing the use of ergogenic aids by American athletes. If anything, public officials' often repeated insistence on the need to defeat Soviet teams in international contests exerted indirect pressure on U.S. sports officials to turn a blind eye to doping.

In the efforts to define and deal with the problem of doping, a combination of factors discouraged effective policy making and, in so doing, reflected the contradictory ways in which doping was conceptualized. In general, the IOC leadership tended to try to shift responsibility to other organizations in the Olympic governance system. National governments generally did not intervene—or, in the case of the Soviet bloc, actively promoted the use of performance enhancement. In the absence of state regulatory involvement, Avery Brundage couched the problem of doping in the context of limited resources and competing policy problems; it was an economic and organization threat. De Merode conceptualized the problem as one of public health and judicial fairness. As these competing definitions were debated over the course of the decade, the larger currents of the Cold War, coupled with a wide availability—and public acceptance—of pharmaceuticals, added another layer to the conceptualization of performance enhancement. If Knud Jensen's death suggested a problem that required swift and effective resolution, Communist-bloc dominance in sport suggested the need for Western officials to fight fire with fire.

Two

TESTING BEGINS

1968 GRENOBLE WINTER GAMES

Leading up to the 1968 Winter and Summer Games, the IOC medical commission tried to exclude the other members of the Olympic governance system from the issue of doping, including the remainder of the IOC. In so doing, de Merode hoped to establish his group as the sole regulatory authority regarding performance enhancement in Olympic competition. The medical commission asserted that the multilayered system of tests proposed for the Winter Games, which included thin-layer chromatography, gas chromatography, "plus any other methods which could prove to be necessary . . . will be given to the IOC Medical Commission only[,] who will decide on any possible further action." Moreover, after two samples had been tested, "no protests will be considered." As for the set of penalties that would be applied in the event of a positive test, the medical commission concluded that in individual sports, athletes found to be using performance-enhancing substances should be removed from the Games, while in team sports, the entire squad "of an athlete who has been shown to have used doping is excluded, *if the team can benefit from this usage.*"[1]

Once the national Olympic committees and international federations were informed of the steps to be taken, however, a significant problem arose in terms of interpreting the commission's definition of doping. Alcohol use was classified as doping, but, as British Olympic Association officer Sandy Duncan noted in a December 1967 letter to Avery Brundage, the athlete's entry sheet required a prospective Olympian to declare "that he has never indulged in an alcoholic drink, nor does he have the intention of so doing."[2] Duncan complained that signing such an oath would be "utterly untrue and makes the competitors' Declaration Form suspect." He also criticized the athletes' entry sheet for its vagueness: "Although details of Olympic Amateurism are set out on the reverse side of the Declaration Form," Duncan wrote, "there are no details of 'dope' so the competitor really doesn't know precisely what he is signing . . . The signing of it in its present form is really making the competitor sign an untruth."[3] In a December 1967 letter to de Merode, USOC physician Daniel Hanley noted that while we "are in accord with your commission that 'doping' is bad . . . it would be most helpful to us if the Medical Commission . . . would state specifically what tests are to be used and how they are to be done." These should include "scientific descriptions so that all nations may then standardize . . . the tests the same way . . . including what levels are to be considered positive."[4]

This request for standardization of a testing protocol under the aegis of the medical commission, however, turned out to be overly ambitious. In preliminary discussions held earlier that year, there was significant reason to believe that the transition to a standardized system would be relatively straightforward. In July 1967, Pedro Ramírez Vásquez, an officer of the organizing committee of the Mexico City Games, had written to Brundage to inform him that he had received the IOC doping resolutions. Vásquez noted that the Mexican organizing committee would "be glad to take steps to put in force all the necessary . . . doping control measures referred to in the [regulations]."[5] Meanwhile, however, the IOC had by October 1967 returned to its belief that the international federations should have an active role in the development of doping policies. It remains uncertain whether this change in approach was an acknowledgment of the political realities of the Olympic governance structure or a reemergence of Brundage's antipathy toward centralized control of doping policies in the IOC. Writing to the international federations, J. W. Westerhoff, IOC secretary general, explained that "we are convinced that only through close co-operation with the International Federations will it be possible for us to find reasonable solutions to these very controversial problems." The IOC, he went on, "would therefore like to ask you to aid us through your experience and inform us if your Federation has any rules on this subject, and if so, what methods you employ . . . We would be very happy to know under what conditions you have worked and what results were obtained."[6]

De Merode remained committed to centralized regulatory control within the medical commission, however. At two IOC executive board meetings in January 1968, de Merode delineated the testing procedures that were to be used at the Winter Games in Grenoble; in his report on prohibited substances, he again excluded anabolic steroids.[7] Although at the time de Merode gave no reason for the exclusion, a statement he made several years later indicates his thinking: "There had been considerable progress in the field of hormones and steroids but it was not possible at this point to control these substances. As the Commission had to be certain before carrying out tests, these products were not on the list of prohibited products."[8] In other words, the inclusion of a pharmacological agent that could not be detected might undermine the legitimacy of the emerging anti-doping framework.

The penalties to be imposed were clarified at an IOC general session meeting held just prior to the opening of the Games.[9] President Brundage later recalled that the federations strongly objected to the proposed anti-doping measures and "hinted that this was a technical matter that should be in their hands."[10] In any event, of the samples taken, according to a post-Games report by Dr. Jacques Thiebault, not one prohibited substance was detected.[11] As the year went on, it became apparent that the IOC's reluctance to take action stemmed from fear of the possible repercussions of a vigorous and efficacious testing system. At an executive board meeting in September 1968, Brundage stated that the limited steps he had taken with regard to the issue were "with the aim of protecting the Medical Commission and the IOC legally." It was agreed that the medical commission should only "go on with its work of supervising but not operating the tests which are to be made only on the written request of IF's [International Federations]."[12]

Early testing efforts were thus characterized by difficulties with definitions and practices, as well as a struggle between de Merode's medical commission and the rest of the Olympic movement, where de Merode pushed for centralization and Brundage, Westerhoff, and the federations consistently tried to "share the wealth." As in 1966, anabolic steroids were again not included on the list of prohibited substances.

GENDER TESTING

During the 1960s, worries about performance-enhancing drugs were coupled with longstanding fears concerning non-females competing as women at the Games.[13] The concern about gender began in the 1936 "Nazi" Olympic Games, when German officials, having been challenged by Polish journalists, did a "sex check" (which was passed) on the American sprinter Helen Stevens. Suspicions about "sex cheating" arose again during the Cold War, when a German man named Herman Ratjen disclosed that Nazi officials had forced him to compete as a woman at the 1936 Games, where he placed fourth in the high jump; "Dora," as he was called, later set a women's world record in the event.[14]

In a 1961 issue of the IOC *Bulletin,* it was proclaimed that although the Olympic movement was beginning to address the problem of doping, "no mention was [made] of a particularly revolting form of doping[,] that of women athletes who take male hormones which lead to castration of the functional cycle of women and amount sometimes to an atrophy of the ovaries which may cause a chronic disease in the long run."[15] In 1967, IOC publications editor Monique Berlioux claimed that gender doping was occurring through certain techniques whereby "the woman's menstruation is stopped by means of medicinal substances. In addition, injections of male hormones are given and these have the twofold effect of increasing physical resistance and of fortifying the muscular tones." Although such steps could not, according to Berlioux, change one's gender, "from then on," she wrote, "certain secondary masculine characteristics may begin to appear."[16]

The IOC executive board discussed gender verification at its October 1966 meeting in Mexico City. At this point, it was decided that delegates at the impending Olympic general session should contemplate, as with drug analyses, the possibility of administering sex tests. Such tests had already been implemented by the International Association of Athletics Federations (IAAF), the world governing body for track and field.[17] Brundage wrote to Arthur Porritt, at that time still head of the IOC anti-doping subcommittee: "In view of the sex developments at the recent European Championships in Budapest and the action of the I.A.A.F., should we not have something in our rules on this subject[?] Will you be good enough to prepare a suggestion for the coming Session in Teheran[?]"[18] Porritt responded, "I can see difficulties in trying to make this comprehensive for all sports. As for a rule on the subject, even with my medical knowledge I would find this a little difficult to compose!" Falling back on the IOC's traditional penchant for avoiding responsibility in scientific matters, he proposed that "it would seem that such individual Federations as had an interest in the subject might follow the good example of the I.A.A.F. and that the I.O.C. might reasonably keep out of this very contentious field."[19] Several of the federations, however, were equally apathetic; IOC member Lord Killanin (a future president of the committee) later recalled that the International Amateur Swimming Federation pragmatically "stood out for a long time against tests, asserting that swimsuits clearly disclose the sex of the competitor."[20]

In Tehran, Porritt said that "the problems of doping, sex tests and anabolic steroids" required "that contacts should be taken up with the Organizing Committee for the Olympic Games so as to make sure that medical machinery to cope with these problems would be available."[21] For the

Grenoble Winter Olympics, the medical commission, "bearing in mind the high cost of these tests and the facilities of the laboratories," as well as hoping to avoid a public relations catastrophe, "suggested testing one female athlete in five, in such a way as to assure ourselves of these facts and avoid unnecessary scandal."[22] Media reports framed the gender issue as an alarming threat to the purity of sport, and athletics policymakers worried, as they did with doping, that inaction might ignite a storm of public criticism. Writing to de Merode in November 1967, USOC chief medical officer Daniel Hanley asserted that "like you, we feel that the publicity which has been given to both of these programs [doping and gender cheating] is unfortunate and we appreciate your efforts to help prevent future sensational stories about them." Hanley was unclear as to the IOC's understanding of gender orientation, and he requested "that the Medical Commission state clearly and in advance their definition of a 'female' and of a 'male' . . . The interpretation of these studies is subject to human error and the Buccal smear techniques [to be used] are not the most accurate."[23]

Given the highly personal nature of sex testing, the medical commission was also concerned with the well-being of the athletes, some of whom, it was felt, might have been unaware of their true chromosomal gender pattern. It therefore proposed that "in the event of some irregularity being found, the result of the control will be given only to the responsible medical officer of the team concerned, and to the President of the IOC Medical Commission or his representative."[24] De Merode, as chair of the medical commission, clarified that "in view of the expense involved, only fifty out of two hundred and fifty female athletes would be tested." De Merode asked for, and received, "the support of the Executive Board in trying to persuade the Organizing Committee [of the Games] to have more athletes tested, if possible all of them." Aware of the delicate nature of the issue, the IOC membership resolved that each female Olympian would be tested through chromosomal analysis of buccal smears and concluded that "the control will be carried out before the Games in such a way as to preserve secrecy and avoid all embarrassment."[25] In buccal examinations, scrapes are taken from an individual's inner cheek; the smears are then scrutinized through a microscope to determine the competitor's chromosomal pattern.[26] For their part, the international federations asked that no sex tests be administered in their respective sports without their prior approval.[27]

At the conclusion of the Winter Olympics in Grenoble, Dr. Jacques Thiebault presented a report describing the activities of the medical commission. Although no abnormalities had been detected among the women examined, several moral and practical issues arose that required the IOC's consideration. The competition, according to Dr. Thiebault, was "the first time that such steps were carried out within the framework of the Olympic Games, which explains certain shortcomings when they were put into practice." However, Thiebault optimistically noted, "these should be easily rectified in the future." In fact, Thiebault had argued before the Games against gender testing out of a belief that "these people are to be pitied, for throughout their lives they will be inadapted [sic] and thanks to sport, they probably tried to achieve a difficult assimilation into an often hostile, and even stupid society." He continued, "These examinations must be carried out in the most absolute medical secrecy, and the more or less radical sporting measures which may follow must be based on the wish, not to harm, but rather to help. Our idea will therefore never be that of punishing, but always that of dissuasion."[28]

Equally important in terms of the image of the Olympic movement, Thiebault asserted that "it is useless to discuss at great length the reasons which crystallized this question; most of the press and unfortu[n]ately the scandal-rags, have for a large part made themselves the echo of these so-called women, built like navvies [sic] and breaking records." He continued, "Already at the European Athletics Championships the Federation carried out checks which were rewarded by a public scandal, which proves that in this sort of thing, *discretion is at least as important as examination techniques.*"[29] As such, the "scandal[s] ensuing from the discovery of a false sex [at the Olympic Games] would inevitably have given rise to a host of juicy headlines and bad taste in the international scandal-rags."[30] Although Thiebault was careful to distinguish his points concerning sex testing from rules prohibiting the use of performance-enhancing drugs, which were, according to Thiebault, "evident attempt[s] at fraud," his emphasis on the voraciousness of the press and the consequent need for discretion became a fixture of Olympic doping policy.

1968 MEXICO CITY OLYMPIC GAMES

After the 1968 Winter Games, a power struggle ensued within the IOC that pitted President Brundage and his followers against the medical commission, few of whose members were attached to the IOC, over the development of doping policy. Brundage held that the international federations should have primary responsibility for anti-doping policy and the medical commission should have only secondary responsibility. De Merode challenged this view. Writing to General Clark Flores at the Mexico City organizing committee, Brundage asserted that "it has never been our idea that the IOC would take permanent charge of the actual testing. This is a technical requirement that rests with the International Federations and is not our province." He concluded, "It was never the intention of the IOC to assume permanently the duty of carrying out these tests anymore than it handles the starting or the timing of the races. The actual testing must remain in the hands of the International Federations."[31]

Brundage also contacted de Merode: "I have been dealing with this matter for twenty years and I am positive that the IOC had *never* had any intention whatsoever of undertaking such an enormous task . . . Our responsibility," Brundage emphasized, "is to have intelligent regulations, to see that the adequate facilities are provided, and that correct methods are used, and that is all. I am sorry that you were not properly informed."[32] In a painstaking analysis of the Olympic medical structure and priorities, Brundage absolved the IOC of even these limited duties. "You will note," he asserted to de Merode and the executive board, "that the testing is to be made by the medical authorities of the Organizing Committee with the assistance of officials of the F.I.M.S." Brundage added, "It was never, never, never intended that the IOC itself should take responsibility for testing . . . We are not equipped for that sort of an operation, ignoring the expense involved."[33] Soon thereafter, Brundage released a circular letter to the various organizations of the Olympic movement outlining the IOC's stance toward testing: "This is a technical matter that must be handled by the International Federations and the National Olympic Committees . . . in co-operation with the Organizing Committee." The IOC and its medical commission, in contrast, played only consultative roles in that they "are ready to advise any [of the aforementioned organizations] . . . which may desire, in pursuing this subject, the benefit of their studies and their experience."[34]

De Merode replied that "the absolute confusion that this statement has caused in everybody's minds is a serious blow to the work we are trying to achieve. This change of opinion brings us back to the question of how much we can depend on the decisions of the I.O.C." Brundage's meddling with previous decisions regarding the medical commission's power should, de Merode continued, be considered "an abuse of authority and would be a serious mortgage on the work we would have liked to foresee in the future . . . I must also add that these extremely delicate matters concern the moral responsibility of the I.O.C. and go far beyond technical questions, if we still wish to remain loyal to the fundamental principles of the Olympic spirit." In the interests of the Olympic movement, however, de Merode hoped that he and Brundage could patch their relationship. He concluded, "I am sure that our next talks in Mexico will help to smooth out these differences of opinion which are certainly only on the surface."[35]

As this conflict trickled down to the other organizations in the Olympic system of governance, confusion ensued as to how the drug tests in Mexico City would be conducted. General José de J. Clark Flores wrote to Brundage complaining of medical commission member Dr. Eduardo Hay's insistence that the IOC controlled the doping protocol. "I have tried to explain to him," Clark Flores stated, "that matters of a technical nature, such as the use of dope by the athletes or the sex tests, are beyond the competence of the IOC. On the contrary, these problems are completely in the line of the International Federations' concern." In terms of a specific procedure, Clark Flores stressed that "these tests would be effected upon request from the International Federations themselves whose demands, as we know, are quite varied and differ a lot one from another."[36] Writing to Pedro Vásquez, chair of the Mexico City Games organizing committee, Brundage confirmed that "this testing will not be done by the International Olympic Committee directly. Facilities would have to be provided by the Organizing Committee . . . [while the] actual testing will be under control of the International Federations concerned."[37]

Aware of the potential for internal IOC strife to erode the effectiveness and prestige of the Olympic movement, Brundage, though still insistent that the IOC keep a low profile with regard to doping, later sought to make amends with de Merode. Cabling de Merode, who was then in Brussels, Brundage, in a rare admission of fault, expressed "regret [over the] misunderstanding on Medical Commission. Perhaps I did not make myself clear." Brundage went on to misrepresent his prior statements on the issue, stating that he could not "understand confusion since all testing in Mexico must be done under its [the medical commission's] supervision as planned before[.] The only difference is testing will be done only at the written request of the International Federations."[38] Later that day, Brundage penned an even more conciliatory letter, stating that "there has been no intention whatsoever on my part to undermine the Medical Commission, which everyone has agreed has accomplished its task with outstanding success." As for the protocol at the Games, Brundage assured de Merode that although the international federations must request drug tests, "if there is any testing in Mexico, it will be done under the supervision of this Commission and according to its regulations and procedures."[39]

The international federations, of course, were no more eager to assume control over the drug tests than Brundage. On September 16, 1968, Brundage received a telegram from a group of European national Olympic committees and international federations congratulating the medical commission on the successful drug regime in Grenoble and expressing their "hope that the I.O.C. will give it full powers to continue these tests in collaboration with the International Federations at the Olympic Games."[40] The Olympic drug control efforts during the 1960s were thus developed within an environment in which no organizational entity, with the exception of the IOC medical commission, wished to assume a position of leadership. De Merode accepted Brundage's apology, promised to work closely with the international federations on technical matters, and assured him that the medical commission sought only "to carry out resolutely adaptable and humanely acceptable tests which are in accordance with the dignity of the Olympic Games." He did warn Brundage, however, that "by tolerating exceptions or only partially putting legislation into force, we would risk being accused of biased opinions and it would seem a flagrant injustice" to the athletes.[41]

With the power struggle thus resolved, Brundage allowed medical commission member Dr. Eduardo Hay to direct the gender verification and drug testing at the Games. The IOC president's previous insistence upon the international federations' taking primary responsibility for implementing such activities derived, according to the minutes of a pre-Games IOC executive board meeting, from concerns that the committee should distance itself from policies that could result in damaging litigation. At an IOC executive board meeting in Mexico City, Brundage asserted that his position "was with the aim of protecting the Medical Commission and the IOC legally." De Merode asserted that the thorny nature of the doping issue required extensive involvement by the medical commission. "It goes without saying," he argued, "that such a complicated mechanism could not be left to different individual Sports Federations and therefore it has been centralized."[42]

At the Mexico City Games, the different international sport organizations cooperated in executing the testing protocol; the medical commission met regularly with officials from the international federations and national Olympic committees at the hotel housing the IOC delegation. "This arrangement," according to a post-Games report by Hay, "greatly facilitated the coordination and the completion of the work." A total of 803 female Olympians submitted to buccal scrapings, which were examined to determine their chromosomal pattern. Only two required clarification by a "Modified Guard Method"; all were confirmed as females. Once the athletes' female sex was confirmed, they received a certificate absolving them of any responsibility to submit to additional verifications at future events sponsored by the IOC.[43]

Hay and the medical commission also directed the doping control procedures, sending "brigades" of technicians out to the individual events to collect urine and blood specimens. In each case, the athletes were provided "notice to report to the office in which the specimens were to be taken," allowing, in one case, "several hours before the athlete was able to provide the specimen." In all, 670 urine samples were examined for various stimulants through a dual-layered technique that included both chromatography in gaseous phase and chromatography on paper; in addition, forty-eight analyses for alcohol were conducted through blood samples.[44]

Even though only two confirmed positive indications of amphetamines were found, Dr. Hay reported that a disturbing number of unknown chemicals were found in the examinations. "It was evident in the analyses," he explained, "that a large number of the samples analyzed contained abnormal products. Analytically, they produce results very similar to some of the drugs commonly used but whose chemical make-up . . . does not correspond to that of the products classified [as prohibited substances]."[45] Remarking upon this problem, an anonymous American weightlifter at the Games wryly asserted: "What ban? Everyone used a new one [performance-enhancing drug] from West Germany. They couldn't pick it up in the test they were using."[46] Hay noted that "if a technique . . . is established as official, it is relatively easy to administer drugs that cannot be identified." He recommended that rather than focusing on specific substances, the IOC should concentrate on a broader definition of doping so that "a positive result may be obtained even though the chemical product is not specified, but rather the group to which the product belongs."[47]

The Olympic movement's tentative first steps toward testing for drugs and chromosomal sex patterns were thus characterized by a confluence of factors that resulted in marginal progress. Chief among these factors was the struggle between IOC president Avery Brundage and IOC medical commission head Alexandre de Merode. Throughout the decade, Brundage worked to shift responsibility for testing to the federations, sometimes arguing that such "technical matters" were not the concern of the IOC, and other times arguing that he wanted to protect the IOC from the potential litigation and scandal associated with doping and men competing as women. De Merode forcefully argued the opposite case, asserting that the only way to conduct a fair and consistent testing program was to centralize responsibility in the IOC medical commission. De Merode prevailed, at least to some extent—though the first attempts to test athletes were plagued by technical problems wherein the specifically banned substances were not found, but the blood samples indicated anomalies associated with drugs of the same class. As the anonymous American weightlifter at the 1968 Mexico City Games declared, "When they get a test for that one, we'll find something else. It's like cops and robbers."[48]

The proliferation of drugs at the Games caused significant concern over the future of the Olympic movement. The ethical dilemma posed by doping even called into question conventional notions of sport as a "pure" exception to the compromising realities of everyday life.[49] As put by *Sports Illustrated* columnist Bil Gilbert in a 1969 retrospective concerning the previous decade, "The use of drugs—legal drugs—by athletes is far from new, but the increase in drug usage in the last 10 years is startling. It could, indeed, menace the tradition and structure of sport itself."[50] Such a pessimistic—and, in hindsight, prescient—analysis should have captivated the attention of both government authorities and private sports administrators, but in the end, it failed to do so. As we will see, the situation at the end of the 1970s would be little better than the state of Olympic doping policy at the time of Gilbert's article.

In the 1970s, a broadening of nationalist forces brought an additional source of pressure on anti-doping policy in Olympic governance. Since its inception in the late nineteenth century, the Olympic movement had been marked by a curious intermingling of nationalist elements alongside a broader internationalist mission.[1] The father of the modern Olympics, Baron Pierre de Coubertin, believed, for instance, that nationalism should maintain a prominent place in Olympic competition. Indeed, as long as nationalism functioned properly, it was for him "by no means detrimental." In de Coubertin's vision, a global institution of athletics would operate as an agent of world peace not by eradicating nationalism, but by incorporating its elements in a "sincere internationalist" framework.[2] De Coubertin warned, however, that unrestrained nationalism in athletics might lead to jingoism, which, in his words, would "[open] the door to all kinds of dangerous misunderstandings and illusions."[3] Over the years, events gave substance to this warning as ultranationalist, politically motivated manipulations of international sport became increasingly apparent features of the Olympic movement. Governmentally sponsored doping was an important element in these developments.

By 1970, the IOC had realized that the widespread use of performance-enhancing substances at the Games was evolving into a dangerous, and increasingly public, ethical crisis. The minutes of an IOC general session in May of that year thus declared that in the 1968 Games and in "more recent cases of deviations from the regulations and moral standards, the question of doping raises the need for energetic and more organised steps in this sensitive sphere of sport and humanism."[4] Medical commission chair Alexandre de Merode, recognizing that "the intensity of international competitions had grown in all Olympic sports," accordingly called for a "well organised and systemical doping control . . . for the Olympic Games."[5] As in the 1960s, de Merode's call for action was met with resistance others in from the Olympic movement. USOC officials, for instance, sought to circumvent doping regulations after what they felt was an unfair suspension of American swimmer Rick DeMont for using an asthma medication approved by a team doctor. More dangerously, the German Democratic Republic, committed to success in elite international sport as an indicator of national vitality, implemented a pervasive state-sponsored doping system in 1975 that would eventually force some 10,000 athletes—many against their will or without their knowledge—to ingest or otherwise absorb potentially harmful performance-enhancing drugs.[6]

At first glance, the intensification of nationalism in international sport at this time seems curious given the lessening of Cold War tensions produced by détente. It might be argued, though, that athletic competitions serve as psychological substitutes for armed conflict during periods of relative international tranquility. Thus, the use of performance-enhancing drugs by athletes at Olympic competitions may have served as a nonmilitary means of waging Cold War battles. As George Orwell observed in 1945, "Serious sport . . . is war minus the shooting."[7] Early hopes that an effective governance structure could exist outside the regulatory influence of nation-states fell short, with countries refraining from involvement in doping policies only out of self-interest. By avoiding controls over performance-enhancing substances enacted by Olympic officials, nations on both sides of the Iron Curtain engaged in what amounted to a pharmacological arms race.

Given the larger political context, it is not surprising that the IOC retreated to its earlier position that it, too, should remain relatively aloof from doping regulation, ceding responsibility to the federations. In 1969, thus, the IOC executive board was unanimous in its applause for the efforts of the IOC medical commission at the Mexico City Games, but "considered that [doping policy and its jurisdiction] should be limited to the period immediately preceeding [sic] and following the Olympic Games."[8] The international federations supported this position, and they were quite willing, as stated by French IOC delegate Comte Jean de Beaumont, to "have the responsibility of carrying out these tests."[9] The executive board, continuing Brundage's restrictive position of the 1960s regarding IOC doping authority, declared that the medical commission would thereafter be limited to a supervisory role while the international federations would be "responsible for carrying out their own dope, alcohol and sex tests . . . [and] the Organizing Committees will provide all facilities."[10] This retreat from centralized responsibility would prove critical in the 1970s as nationalistic forces overwhelmed the capacities of a de facto leaderless, organizationally diffused Olympic policy response.

Brundage, still engaged in a somewhat prickly relationship with de Merode, continued to discourage a robust regulatory response by the IOC. Writing to de Merode in May 1971, he suggested that "it would be wise for your Commission to make a contact [sic] with the Federations which have had the most experience with the necessity for [drug] control." Referring to the set of doping regulations to be implemented at the upcoming 1972 Munich Olympic Games, he wrote, "If they approve the regulations that you finally adopt, it will add strength and power to them."[11] Brundage seemed to support de Merode's policy initiatives, but he also (once again) called for de Merode to defer to the federations.

Brundage also brought financial arguments to bear on his longstanding position that doping policy should not be centralized in de Merode's medical commission. Having been informed by IOC information director Monique Berlioux of two medical commission conferences for which the expenses would be "tremendous," Brundage responded that "there is no use wasting a lot of money on these superfluous meetings if we can avoid it."[12] After learning that the Munich Games organizing committee would pay the costs of the sessions, Brundage underscored his conviction that the foundation of IOC doping policy should center on delegation of responsibility. In a note to de Merode, he wrote, "It is a little embarrassing to have others pay the expenses, but probably in this instance it is not out of order seeing that it is one of the obligations of the Organizing Committee to prepare for the medical tests."[13]

De Merode and his commission pressed on. At the July 29, 1971, meeting of the medical commission, discussions focused on a new doping control brochure, 4,000 copies of which were to be distributed to the various members of the Olympic establishment. Presenting the idea to the IOC leadership in September of that year, de Merode expressed confidence "that the application of these presented methods of control, and their publication, will have a positive effect in the immediate decrease and future elimination of the danger of doping in modern sport."[14] The brochure carefully divided the responsibility for testing between the medical commission and the federations. As for the actual authority over drug controls, the international federations would have the "technical responsibility for sports matters (number of checks, persons to be examined, times)," while the medical commission would have the "moral responsibility for the different kinds of controls and [would] supervise their organization." Further, guilty athletes could only be "eliminated from the Olympic Games by the International Federation concerned following the proposal of the IOC Medical Commission."[15] The minutes from a 1972 medical commission meeting noted that the international federations were wary of taking responsibility for testing, asserting that it was "generally agreed that it should be the Medical Commission who carried out the control."[16]

Meanwhile, President Brundage, having heard that methods to identify anabolic steroids were under development, asked de Merode whether the medical commission "had found any [definitive] method of detecting [such] hormones," which were quickly replacing amphetamines as elite athletes' drugs of choice.[17] Such tests, he had been told, were problematic in that anabolic steroids were untraceable if the athlete ceased their administration several weeks prior to the Games.[18] The IOC executive board nevertheless limited the medical commission's authority to the "period immediately preceeding [sic] and following the Olympic Games."[19] De Merode explained that the world's leading expert on the subject, Dr. Arnold Beckett of Great Britain, "had not gone far enough in his research for the Medical Commission to use any control in this field."[20] The early 1970s were thus marked by IOC deferral of responsibility to the federations and IOC restriction of medical commission authority, rendering Olympic regulatory policies especially vulnerable to the burgeoning nationalistic forces of the decade.

1972 SAPPORO WINTER OLYMPIC GAMES

Several national Olympic committees echoed the sentiments of the federations, seeking greater uniformity in regulations and centralization of authority for anti-doping policy. The Belgian national committee, for example, submitted a proposal, subsequently rejected by the IOC, "to entrust a [new] Commission to study the drafting of some simple rules, which could be applied in all cases, for every sportsman and every sportswoman and of which they can avail themselves in every country, for every sport."[21] And Dr. Daniel Hanley, USOC chief medical officer, addressed the USOC board of directors as follows: "Dope control is becoming a very strong issue, and I think we should formulate some policy . . . I think we can ignore it, if you want to . . . but, more and more, many individuals and some important segments of our society, like the press, are looking to you for direction."[22] Indeed, in 1973 the U.S. Senate held hearings on drug use by athletes. U.S. Olympian Harold Connolly testified that "the overwhelming majority of the international track and field athletes I have known would take anything and do anything short of killing themselves to improve their athletic performance."[23]

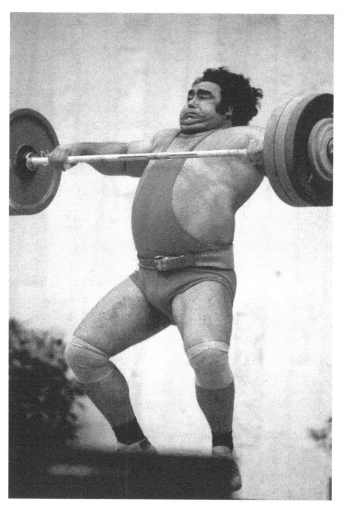

FIGURE 3.   *Vasily Alexeyev in action during weightlifting event at the 1980 Summer Olympics in Moscow (Jerry Cooke/Sports Illustrated/Getty Images).*

This reported willingness to "take anything" was not limited to track and field. U.S. weightlifter Ken Patera, after winning a gold medal in the 1971 Pan-American super-heavyweight weightlifting contest, asserted his eagerness for a rematch with the Soviet Union's Vasily Alexeyev, who had defeated him in the previous year's World Championships in Columbus, Ohio. Patera openly claimed, "Last year, the only difference between me and him was that I couldn't afford his drug bill. Now I can. When I hit Munich next year, I'll weight in at about 340, maybe 350 [pounds]. Then we'll see which are better—his steroids or mine."[24] As for any response by American sport officials, Patera later recalled that he "didn't hear a peep out of anyone from the U.S. Olympic Committee."[25] Although Patera was not reprimanded by the body, he was a topic of discussion in its deliberations. Dr. Hanley, speaking in October 1971 before the USOC board of directors, apologized "for that mental pigmy we had aboard, who sounded off and shot his mouth off, afterward, about subjects he knew absolutely nothing about."[26] Hanley's remarks underscore the continuing inability of the Olympic movement to face the scope of the doping problem.

At the 1972 Winter Olympic Games in Sapporo, Japan, tests were administered to 211 athletes. These tests detected only one instance of doping (a West German hockey player named Alois Schloder), an astonishingly low number given such public testimonials as that of Patera.[27] Of course, the dearth of positive tests was due in significant measure to the absence of steroid screening. Several additional issues emerged during the Sapporo Games that would have significant effects for the IOC's medical policies. Schloder's membership in a team sport sparked significant controversy in terms of how to address instances in which doping affected more than an individual. The relevant IOC regulation in effect at the time stated that "if the athlete belongs to a team, the game or competition in question shall be forfeited by that team," and, it continued, "a team in which one or more members have been found guilty of doping may be disqualified from the Olympic Games."[28] In a post-Games IOC meeting, however, de Merode stated that "this rule had not been applied in Sapporo because of technical reasons and the Commission had decided that the rule should not be applied in the future."[29] The West German squad was thus allowed to continue at the games, where it eventually finished seventh.

There was also some debate regarding sex testing. After the Sapporo Games, Danish researchers publicly questioned the efficacy of the Olympic gender verification regime, which was based on the identification of an individual's chromosomal—rather than somatic and/or psychosocial—sex.[30] Prior to the Games, Dr. Ingborg Bausenwein, a physician who worked with female athletes on the West German Olympic team, had questioned the whole enterprise of sex testing, arguing that before the test's implementation in 1968, "five out of 11 women's world records [in track-and-field] were held by hermaphrodites."[31] The Danish scientists countered that "the decision of the international Olympic committee to demand that all female competitors at the Olympic games should be 'sex-tested' with the aim of excluding sex chromatin negative individuals from competing with females is open to criticism for scientific as well as for medical and ethical reasons."[32]

Several months later, Brundage sought the opinion of the IOC medical commission, writing to de Merode that "I am happy I didn't realise [sic] all the complications when I was 25, but seriously this is very disquieting and must have the attention of your committee." In a notable display of humor from the usually acerbic IOC president, Brundage lightly concluded, "Maybe the eye of a 25 year old would be better."[33] The early chromatin tests were criticized mainly because they threatened to shatter the lives of numerous women, most of whom held no significant physiological advantage over their fellow competitors.[34] In the end, the chromatin tests were retained and an alternative system was not put in effect until the 1992 Albertville Winter Olympic Games.[35] Explaining the decision to keep the chromatin tests, de Merode pointed out that the IOC's "practical" concerns outweighed the researchers' "scientific side." Brundage agreed, stating that "the problem of the Danish doctors being purely theoretical was very different from that of the IOC's which was practical."[36]

1972 MUNICH OLYMPIC GAMES

The organizing committee for the 1972 Munich Summer Games was confident about the steps—estimated to cost $669,195—that it was taking with regard to the curtailment of doping at its competitions. In a report to the IOC in early 1972, the Munich organizing committee asserted that "there was good co-operation with the International Federations" in developing a rigorous control system through "uniform guidelines . . . drawn up on a sound scientific basis." The committee further claimed (quite mistakenly, in light of later events) that "the entire question of doping control in Munich has been very well thought out so that mistakes and protest are virtually impossible."[37] The complex regulatory system of the Olympics, in which the IOC, organizing committees, and international federations each played important roles, led to confusion as to possible situations in which drug treatments might be allowable. A 1968 report from the medical board of the International Cycling Union circulated to IOC members prior to the 1972 Munich Games, for instance, concluded that "a certain tolerance may be admitted . . . concerning the [type] of administration, the used dosis [sic], and the therapeutic goals" of selected classes of tranquilizers, sedatives, ephedrine, ether, caffeine, and hormones.[38]

Such ambiguity eventually led to an environment in which, according to an unofficial poll of all track-and-field competitors in Munich by U.S. squad member Jay Silvester, 68 percent of the men used some type of anabolic steroid prior to the competitions.[39] Pat O'Shea, the American weight-lifting team physiologist, likewise claimed that every member of the squad was using some sort of performance-enhancing drug.[40] The problem had become so acute that Dr. John Zeigler, a U.S. team physician during the 1960s, quit. "I found some of the athletes were taking 20 times the recom-mended dosage [of various ergogenic drugs]," he asserted. "I lost interest in fooling with IQ's of that caliber. Now it's about as widespread among these idiots as marijuana."[41]

Such public claims should have been cause for alarm among Ameri-can sport officials, but calls for reform were not forthcoming. In fact, the USOC issued a vehement protest when sixteen-year-old American swim-mer Rick DeMont was stripped of his gold medal, having tested positive for a prohibited stimulant after winning the 400-meter freestyle competi-tion.[42] DeMont later explained that he had awoken early in the morning of September 1, 1972, "wheezing," and had taken three tablets of his asthma medication, Marax, over the next several hours.[43] Although DeMont had cleared his use of Marax, which contains the banned substance ephedrine, with U.S. team physicians, they had apparently made no effort to inform examiners in Munich. After the swimmer's positive test, head U.S. team physician Winston Rhiel wrote to the IOC that DeMont "has a history of bronchial asthma and allergy . . . [and] Mr. DeMont has taken this medi-cine [Marax] on his own at infrequent intervals to control the symptoms." Dr. Rhiel argued that "considering all of the above we do not feel that this young athlete has used any medication for the purposes of enhancing his performance."[44] USOC president Clifford Buck went a step further, argu-ing that "it would be inordinately cruel and undeserving if this young man is punished for following his doctor's instructions in order that he may stay alive. This 16-year-old boy, because he loves his sport, has by persevering will and grueling training, overcome a physical handicap to excel in his sport."[45]

The IOC medical commission took a different position. At first de Me-rode recommended that DeMont be allowed to keep his medal, but he changed his mind, urging the IOC executive board to strip DeMont of the award. De Merode also declared that DeMont would not be permit-ted to participate in additional competitions in Munich, including the 1,500-meter freestyle swim, in which he already held the world record. De Merode further stated that "the persons accompanying the athlete [U.S. team officials] should be punished according to the recommendation of the IOC Medical Commission, since they were clearly co-responsible for the incident."[46] After the executive board confirmed DeMont's suspension,

Brundage asked USOC president Clifford Buck to coordinate the return of DeMont's medal and informed him of the IOC's additional conclusion that "much of the responsibility for this disqualification rests on your team medical authorities, who are severely reprimanded."[47]

The harshness apparent in these words reflected broader frictions between U.S. and international sports leaders. At first glance, Brundage's twenty-year tenure as IOC president seemed to suggest that the United States served as a powerful voice in the international sports community. And, while the country certainly remained influential, U.S. officials increasingly perceived anti-American sentiments among IOC leaders. An array of seemingly biased decisions in Munich seemed to confirm their beliefs, especially a loss by the U.S. basketball team to the Soviet Union after Olympic referees made a controversial call near the end of the contest. On appeal of this decision, the votes of three Communist-bloc members against those of an Italian and a Puerto Rican only confirmed such suspicions. In protest, the members of the U.S. squad refused to accept their silver medals or even participate in the awards ceremony.[48]

In another incident, the IOC blamed the USOC for an alleged "black power salute" by two African American athletes after they finished first and second in the 400-meter sprint. Describing the episode as repeating the notorious protest made by Tommie Smith and Juan Carlos four years earlier, the IOC criticized U.S. team officials for failing to control their athletes. "Being the second time that the USOC had permitted such occurrences on the athletic field," an official IOC communiqué asserted, "these two athletes . . . would, therefore, be eliminated from taking part in any future Olympic competition . . . The United States NOC [National Olympic Committee] has apologized and has been cautioned about future competitions." Reading between the lines of the pronouncement at the Olympic press center in Munich, one observer remarked that

> the language of this extraordinary communiqué suggested to the imagination that [the African American athletes] turned about, lowered their shorts, bent, and "mooned" black asses into the old white face of Avery Brundage. For this, Brundage would punish the American nation.[49]

In yet another Munich scandal, this one involving doping, Wille Grut, secretary general of the Union Internationale de Pentathlon Moderne et Biathlon (UIPMB), was directed by representatives of twenty national Olympic committees to seek the addition of tranquilizers to the IOC's list of prohibited substances.[50] The following day, Grut met with de Merode, representatives of the Munich Games organizing committee, and the chief lab technician for doping tests to officially submit this proposal.[51] As the international federations held primary jurisdiction over such matters at the time, the medical commission agreed to the addition of tranquilizers after it was concluded that the laboratory had enough capacity and the organizing committee would pay for the additional tests.[52] Grut accordingly wrote to Dieter Krickow, the organizing committee member responsible for the modern pentathlon, to confirm the decision, after which Krickow informed the individual teams.[53]

UIPMB officials began to regret their progressive actions, however, when sixteen positive cases of drug use were found through the doping checks.[54] Grut then denied the request for the tests. UIPMB president Sven Thofelt declared that the decision to add tranquilizers to the list had been made without authorization and that the federation had never been informed of any such decision.[55] After the UIPMB representatives were presented with evidence of the events, Grut pled negligence, explaining that "UIPMB did not ever officially ask the IOC Medical Commission to add 'tranquilizers' . . . I should not have allowed a non[-]competent meeting of team captains to charge me to forward their opinion." He concluded, "I now feel that this task has not been one for which I am properly trained . . . I very much regret the loss of time and money I seem to have caused your commission."[56] Brundage queried de Merode about the lack of sanctions, and de Merode released a statement declaring that the "Medical Commission of the IOC must not interfere in the internal affairs of an International Federation and has therefore suspended all further action for the time being."[57]

Given their public castigation by the IOC in the DeMont case, American sports officials considered the excuses as an intolerable slap in the face. USOC president Clifford Buck wrote to IOC member Lord Killanin, who would succeed Brundage as IOC president in 1972, that "it seems most inconsistent that prompt severe action was taken on Mr. DeMont in swimming as well as others and then not take disqualifying action against fourteen found guilty of doping in Modern Pentathlon." He continued, "DeMont is a sixteen year old boy who was taking his normal prescribed medication for a chronic problem and not to enhance his performance, whereas the guilty pentathletes are mature individuals who knowingly and deliberately took a banned drug to improve their performance in competition in violation of a rule of which they were aware." Buck concluded, "In the interest of justice, fair play, the honor and integrity of the Olympic Games, and for all athletes who did not indulge in taking forbidden drugs during the shooting event of Modern Pentathlon, it is respectfully requested that the IOC Executive Board reconsider the decision."[58] Even Brundage noted that the incident was leading to "tremendous opposition" and that in the future "some distinction would have to be made between medicine and doping."[59]

Two additional occurrences also highlighted the problems caused by the inconsistent penalties that derived from ambiguous standards. Although the IOC had decided at the Sapporo Games not to suspend national teams after doping was found among individual squad members, the ruling was contradictorily applied in Munich. Tests confirmed drug use by a Puerto Rican basketball player, but the analyses took so long that the team was allowed to continue play throughout the course of the tournament. In the end, the player was disqualified, but the team was not, and its victories were consequently upheld. The Dutch cycling team's bronze medal, on the other hand, was rescinded after one of its riders tested positive for coramine, a substance prohibited by the IOC but not by the International Cycling Union. During the IOC executive board's deliberations, William Jones, secretary general of the Fédération Internationale de Basketball Amateur, pointed out that while one set of rules "stated that teams were disqualified [only] if the team had benefited from an athlete taking dope . . . the doping brochure . . . said that the team would be disqualified [automatically] if one of the players was found guilty."[60]

Four   OLD PROBLEMS AND
NEW LEADERSHIP

The inconsistent application of doping regulations in conjunction with the Black September terrorist attacks—during which thirteen Israeli Olympians were killed—led to significant introspection among Olympic policymakers in the aftermath of the Munich Games. This introspection coincided with the retirement of Avery Brundage as IOC president. Having ruled for twenty years with an iron grip, Brundage retired with the prediction that the movement would not survive in his absence.[1] Hoping for a less dictatorial leader, the IOC elected Lord Michael Morris Killanin, an Irishman, as its new president. "He was the key element," as later put by sports administrator Alain Coupat, "in the evolution from this totally closed organization under Brundage to the open regime of Samaranch [who succeeded Killanin in 1980]." Unfortunately, Killanin was unsuited to effective leadership in the anti-doping effort. Coupat characterized him as "indecisive."[2] The fact that Killanin was regarded as a transition figure within the movement also bode poorly for the future direction of Olympic doping policy.

In February of 1973, de Merode called for changes in the IOC doping rules. "The experience in Munich," he stated, "had shown the need of having strict regulations and many IFs [international federations] had expressed the wish that the IOC should take a stand." As for the longstanding directive that only competition medalists should be investigated, de Merode argued that "the control of the first three in any event was insufficient." The unequal treatment of the Puerto Rican basketball team and the Dutch cycling squad suggested the need for a uniform policy stating that "if any member of a team was found guilty of doping, the whole team had to be disqualified."[3] Within the USOC, deliberations likewise concentrated on the problems caused by the decentralized doping control system, in which each sport operated under a different set of rules. At an early 1973 committee meeting, USOC official General Hains said, "You've got five conflicting sports . . . There has been no attempt to effect doping control, for riding, for fencing, for shooting, for swimming."[4]

In addition, reports began to circulate that athletes were taking advantage of loopholes within the IOC's list of banned substances by finding new, equally effective compounds to ingest. At a 1973 U.S. Senate hearing, former American Olympian Phillip Shinnick asserted that "new ways to beat the system are devised once new precautions are taken."[5] Rumors swirled that Communist-bloc nations had developed a performance-enhancing formula that combined several vitamins with caffeine and nicotinamide, both of which were unlisted substances. Researching the effects of the formulation on volunteers after the Games, Swiss chemist David James, formerly an American elite sprinter, concluded that the subjects of his study benefited in several ways: "actions were more rapid, it seemed to delay fatigue, their reaction was diminished, their motor activity was better." Although not covered under current IOC rules, a tablespoon of the drug, he concluded, could potentially have as much impact as a standard dose of amphetamine sulfate.[6]

The link between nationalism and doping was striking in these developments. Shinnick, for instance, described an episode during his time as a manager for the U.S. team at a previous World University Games in Budapest. American government officials with the squad constantly reminded the athletes of the need "to win so that we could beat the 'Commies'." Shinnick recalled that "implicit in this value [was] the assumption that the world has one winner and all the rest losers in each event. This type of pressure leads toward drug abuse as clearly as the need for the coach to win to retain his job."[7] Within the Olympic structure, these pressures resulted in conflicts of interest among medical officers in sports organizations. Daniel Hanley, for example, was both a USOC physician and a member of the IOC medical commission, which presented a conflict of interest in the DeMont case. In the aftermath, the IOC established that "no member of the [medical] commission could be a [National] team doctor."[8]

The greatest surge of nationalism, though, came in the form of a clandestine state-sponsored doping regime in the German Democratic Republic (GDR) run by that country's Ministry of State Security—the notorious secret police, popularly known as the Stasi. After the Second World War, East German policymakers worked hard to convince both foreign and domestic audiences that their country should be respected as an independent nation.[9] In their list of possibilities for the pursuit of this goal, these officials considered membership in the Olympic movement a high priority—perhaps second only to a seat at the United Nations. Over time, the desire for mere membership was supplanted by the dream of East German athletes standing atop Olympic medal podiums as global audiences stirred at the first notes of "Auferstanden aus Ruinen," the national anthem. During the 1970s, the East German government developed a training system unrivaled by any other in the world.[10]

With a total population of only 17 million, the country became an athletic superpower with the aid of many of its top scientists; after joining Olympic competition at the 1972 Munich Games, for instance, East German athletes won gold medals at a per capita rate that was roughly fifteen times higher than that of the United States.[11] East German leaders, IOC official Dick Pound stated,

> viewed them [athletes of the GDR] as cold warriors. They were at the Olympics to demonstrate the superiority of their political system. They were servants of the state, with no other purpose. They had been identified and trained at the expense of the state and with all of the resources of the state, and they were expected to perform accordingly. And they were expendable warriors.[12]

After the Cold War, East German athletes sued GDR sports officials; the testimony of club sport instructor Henrich Misersky illustrates the East German characterization of sport as a type of warfare. Recalling a conversation with GDR biathlon coach Kurt Hinze, Misersky outlined the pressure put on him to cooperate in the Stasi program: "When it became clear that I was not going to change my mind, I was personally attacked. Referring to his idea that GDR sport was a 'military affair,' Hinze called me a civilian and accused me of having an incorrect political orientation. He said that people like me were reactionary and had to disappear."[13]

East Germany's nationalist conceptualization of sport reflected both the global ideological struggle between the Communist bloc and the Western world and the East German desire to demonstrate independence from its Soviet masters. Having been formed from the area occupied by the Red Army during the aftermath of the Second World War, the GDR remained economically and politically dependent on the Soviet Union throughout the duration of the Cold War. During policy debates, little tolerance existed for those who disagreed with Moscow's decisions. In an early, revealing demonstration of this relationship, Soviet troops went into action in the summer of 1953 as a response to protests by hundreds of thousands of workers in East Berlin. From that point forward, Soviet officials continu-

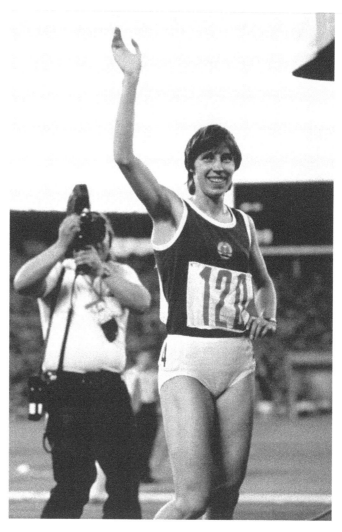

FIGURE 4.   *Marita Koch of the German Democratic Republic smiles as she waves to the crowd after winning the women's 400-meter final at the Summer Olympics in Moscow, July 28, 1980 (STAFF/AFP/Getty Images).*

ally strategized on how to maintain their symbolic authority over the GDR, which served as an exemplar of Soviet power in Eastern Europe.[14]

Soviet sports officials consequently perceived the efforts made by War-saw Pact countries in international sport—and especially those of the GDR—as potential indicators of dissension on the eastern side of the Iron

Curtain. In describing a visit to a Soviet training facility several years after the East German doping system began to produce astonishing successes, sport scientist Ladislav Pataki thus remarked:

> The Soviets were not at all worried about whether or not they could beat American athletes in international competitions. They were certain they could. What worried them was the growing power of other Eastern Bloc countries, including Bulgaria, Romania, Poland, Hungary, Czechoslovakia, and even Cuba, which they also categorized as Eastern Bloc . . . The country that worried them most, however, was East Germany.[15]

A 1973 Stasi report that surfaced in the 1990s documented an "on-off" analysis of Oral-Turinabol (a type of anabolic steroid) in terms of its performance-enhancing effects on forty track-and-field athletes.[16] At the 1968 Mexico City Games, the head of the GDR's doping system, Dr. Manfred Höppner, utilized a protocol that allowed Margitta Gummel to set a new world record in the shot put by throwing 19.61 meters. A fellow contestant, Brigitte Berendonk, later described Gummel at the event: "She was huge. She had massive shoulders and arms. Her body had transformed since the last time we competed. She was clearly a she-man."[17] In Munich—the first Summer Games in which the East Germans competed as a separate team—they built on this initial success, winning a total of sixty-six medals, third best among the competing nations.[18]

East German athletes under the age of eighteen were told that the "little blue pills" they were being given were "vitamins"; those who were older were required to take an oath of silence concerning what were termed "performance-enhancing supplements."[19] The effects of the drugs were stunning; in March 1977, Höppner informed Stasi officials that

> at present anabolic steroids are applied in all Olympic sporting events . . . and by all national teams. The application takes place according to approved basic plans, in which special situations of individual athletes are also considered. The positive value of anabolic steroids for the development of a top performance is undoubted . . . From our experience made so far it can be concluded that women have the greatest advantage from treatments with anabolic hormones . . . Especially high

is the performance-supporting effect following the first administration of anabolic hormones, especially with junior athletes.[20]

For the athletes, anabolic steroids had dangerous side effects. Dr. Ulrich Sunder, chief of the GDR Sports Medical Service, however, "was told by [his] medical superiors that the deep voice and the hair and the virilization would reverse after the women stopped taking them, so we did not worry about long-term consequences." After all, he concluded, everyone was using drugs, including the Western states, "so why should we not compete on that level playing field?"[21]

Unaware of the extent of the GDR's doping regime, the IOC leadership focused on modest steps to improve its doping control system. At a February 1973 IOC executive board meeting, IOC member Comte de Beaumont criticized the practice of handing out medals before the results of the drug tests were known, suggesting that the IOC reverse the order of events. De Merode asserted that implementation of the proposal was impossible: "unless there was a lapse of two or three days before the awarding of medals, this would be out of the question." As a compromise, the medical commission chair agreed that both the initial and confirmation samples could be analyzed at the same time instead of sequentially. He also argued that the IOC's list of banned substances should be reconciled with those of the international federations. "It was unfortunate what had happened in the cycling cases," he noted, referring to the suspension of the Dutch cycling team in Munich, "but the Federation should have adhered to the IOC list." He then called for a meeting between IOC and federation officials before the 1976 Montreal Games to "make sure that all agreed [on] the IOC prohibited list."[22] And, in a post-Brundage assertion of the authority of the medical commission, de Merode made it clear that the international federations should adhere to the IOC's list, rather than the other way around.[23]

By May 1975, the medical commission had made some progress in these areas. In addition, the IOC's list of banned substances was finally updated to include anabolic steroids. This was made possible through the development of several tests reported by scientists in the British medical literature that could detect such chemicals in the human body. As de Merode stated, "The progress of the scientific work proposed gives a complete guarantee as to the accuracy of the results that can be obtained."[24] In July of that year, two articles appeared in a special issue of the *British Journal of Sports*

Medicine outlining alternative analytical techniques. One described the use of radioimmunoassay and the other recommended a combination of gas chromatography and mass spectrometry.[25] Seeking the broadest possible solution, the IOC adopted both techniques; unfortunately, Olympic officials still lacked an accurate test for the natural counterpart of synthetic anabolic steroids: testosterone.[26] This provided a significant loophole for unscrupulous competitors. Dr. Arnold Beckett, member of the IOC medical commission, noted that "some people and some countries are at present overcoming this disadvantage of having to stop [anabolic steroid treatments] before an event by injecting the male hormone testosterone; although this drug can be detected, the fact that this is also an endogenous material means at present we cannot act."[27]

IOC president Lord Killanin lauded the effort as "good news indeed," but the new tests failed to solve several problems.[28] Many performance-enhancing drugs, including anabolic steroids, could be used by athletes during training and then stopped shortly before competition to avoid their detection.[29] In announcing the radioimmunoassay procedure, Dr. Roger Bannister, the world's first sub-four-minute miler, suggested that a successful policy would feature "snap checks" in which specimens would be collected without prior notice and at varying intervals. "Giving these sort of details of timing," he continued, "would be against the interests of what we are trying to do."[30] De Merode and the medical commission, however, remained rooted to the notion that doping analyses should take place only during the Olympic competitions, in part because the tests were so expensive.[31] Referring to the 1976 Montreal Games, de Merode told IOC officials that "the steroids could be detected, provided the last dosage was taken within three weeks before the test. If dosages had been administered more than three weeks before the test, then this could not be detected."[32]

Before the Montreal Games, the new tests for anabolic steroids were used in trial runs at the 1974 British Commonwealth Games in Auckland, and in that year's European Track and Field Championships.[33] In Auckland, nine samples tested positive for anabolic steroids, but no athletes were disqualified, or even named. At the European Championships, Adrian Paulen, president of the European Amateur Athletic Federation, asserted prior to the meet that no punishments would be handed out in that the procedures were for research purposes only.[34] British shot-putter Geoff Capes described the resulting satisfaction among the athletes: "You could hear the sigh of relief as it echoed round the team hostels that the tests would not disqualify us."[35] At the 1975 European [Track-and-Field] Cup, however, two athletes were disqualified from the contest and then suspended by their governing body after tests confirmed their use of anabolic steroids.[36]

1976 MONTREAL OLYMPIC GAMES

In view of the issues concerning anabolic steroids, the IOC medical commission appointed a subcommittee to investigate implementation of the new tests at its July 14, 1976, meeting, which was held only a few days before the official opening of the Games. Several days later, the subcommittee issued a report with a description of the problem, alternative courses of action, and a comprehensive set of recommendations.[37] Chief among the subcommittee's concerns was the IOC's preference that the analyses should be conducted, and their results announced, prior to the events so that athletes who tested positive would not be allowed to compete.[38] The subcommittee noted that "no sample received after the 18th of July 1976 can be analyzed (and rechecked) before the end of the Games"; this was particularly problematic in that although "many samples have already been submitted for analyses . . . it is probable that some . . . designated athletes will not be sampled before the . . . deadline."[39]

An ideal pre-Games testing regimen was therefore impossible given the time constraints involved. The subcommittee pointed out, however, that "no mention is made in the Medical Commission regulations that results have to be made available during the Games . . . It is important to realize that taking action on definitive results from analysis done after the end of the Games is already accepted for regular doping control [i.e., for drugs other than anabolic steroids]." The subcommittee thus suggested that the IOC implement the procedures with the understanding that postcompetition sanctions could be applied. This was the "only action which constitutes a deterrent to competitors against their own foolishness and doctors or coaches against irresponsible actions not in the best interest of competitors."[40] De Merode assured his IOC counterparts that "the Medical Commission would only propose sanctions on athletes if it was absolutely certain . . . If any doubt existed at all, no decision would be taken."[41]

The lack of pre-Games tests at the national level was a problematic aspect of the Olympic doping control framework. Reports began to circulate that many athletes were using performance-enhancing substances to qualify for the Games. Twenty-three American competitors failed the drug control tests at the U.S. Olympic track-and-field trials in Eugene, Oregon; none were punished.[42] After qualifying in the discus, Jay Silvester, who had competed in three previous Olympic Games, stated, "I can't ethically accept the use of steroids. But I would have to say that 98 to 99 per cent, no, 100 per cent of the international caliber throwers are taking them." Silvester went on to say that "it would have been a disadvantage to have the control at this meet. None of the European athletes have such a control, so we would have been at a disadvantage."[43]

The IOC tests served several purposes for the USOC, however. Some officials sincerely believed that the tests could help dampen the use of performance-enhancing substances by their competitors. Other USOC officials thought that the testing would give American athletes the opportunity to learn the ins and outs of the Olympic testing protocol. As stated by USOC member Bob Giegenbach, "It has been widely advertised and agreed upon that, in the final Olympic trials for men and women in Track and Field, that [sic] we will duplicate the doping procedure to be used at Montreal."[44] In a letter to USOC physician Daniel Hanley, Kenneth Bender and Dr. Dean Lockwood informed him that a large number of American swimmers had tested positive in precompetition testing and suggested that "all competitors in future competition be . . . advised on . . . detection procedures."[45]

During the Games, a total of 1,800 urine specimens were collected in "conventional" testing procedures for prohibited drugs; three positive drug indications were obtained. In the new anabolic steroid screens, eight instances of anabolic steroid use were identified among the 275 tests for such substances.[46] Among those testing positive for anabolic steroids were two American weightlifters, Mark Cameron and Phil Grippaldi, both of whom were suspended.[47] Remembering their experience with DeMont, USOC officials protested that they were "shocked and appalled in having to learn of penalties enforced by the [IOC] Medical Commission in the case of Mark Cameron."[48] They were, in addition, infuriated by what they perceived to be several mistakes within the drug control procedures. USOC president Philip Krumm stated, "We seriously question the validity of the procedures used and the random selection of subjects which resulted in inequities in the pre-competition testing for steroids." Taking issue with the inability of his athletes to recognize the loopholes within the procedures, he complained that the controls "were not clearly enunciated prior to the Games, or prior to the arrival of the various squads." Equally shocking, Krumm continued, was the fact that the penalties had been released to the public before the USOC was informed.[49]

American sport officials were not alone in such criticisms. Boleslaw Kapitan, president of the Polish Olympic committee, wrote to Killanin that "we deplore the fact that the medical tests were so prolonged." Kapitan claimed that his federation learned of the positive test result for Zbigniew Kaczmarek, a Polish weightlifter, seven days after the closing ceremonies and three weeks after he had received a gold medal. More importantly, Kapitan asserted, "The publication of the results of the medical tests in the international press before the IOC had announced its decision and probably contrary to your intentions, is prejudicial to the essential interests of sport." As for the validity of the procedures that were used, Kapitan's medical consultants informed him that several of the seals used in the specimen containers were defective; they could easily be opened and their contents changed. "Under these circumstances, since our athlete categorically denies having used Dianabol and as the identification of the contents of the bottles is extremely dubious, . . . we feel obliged to deny the regularity of the way in which the medical tests were carried out."[50]

Warned by IOC doping expert Arnold Beckett that "some countries may endeavour to make a political issue of this and challenge the efficacy of the tests," Killanin sought to dispel questions concerning the validity of the doping protocols by authorizing an article in the IOC *Olympic Review*.[51] Killanin was concerned about the premature release of information about the test results; he wrote that "[I] am most interested to know the first 'leak' . . . I am interested to know whether at any time an 'IOC Spokesman' was referred to in the [press] cuttings."[52] Several days later, the IOC medical commission released a statement saying that it "deplores the publication of names of competitors before analysis of the second samples of urines had confirmed the presence of a steroid. The information concerning names and countries involved was not released by the commission."[53] After the Games, de Merode blamed other members of the international sport community, speculating that the "leakage might have come from the then Secretary General of the [International Weightlifting Federation]."[54] The IOC medical commission defended the suspensions, stating that "while points of protest were heard about the procedure . . . after due consideration, we reject these protests on the ground that the agreed procedure had been followed and there was no evidence of violation of security."[55]

LEGACY OF THE 1976 MONTREAL GAMES

American competitors were angered by the fact that not a single athlete from the GDR competing at the Games was included on the list of disqualified individuals. Watching the women's swimming events, Rod Strachan, the gold medalist in the 400-meter individual medley, described the incredible physical discrepancy between the American and East German female competitors. "If you look at the East Germans," he asserted, "they don't look exactly like they're girls. They're quite a bit bigger than most of the men on the American team. They could go out for football at U.S.C. They've got some big guys there."[56] Five-time U.S. long jumper Willye White added, "The only way you can tell it's a woman is by their bust." Future American success, according to White, required a cynical incorporation of East German methods: "If we're going to compete against synthetic athletes, we must become syntheti[c] athletes."[57]

In spite of the USOC condemnation of the GDR doping regime, USOC officials approved the formation of a panel, headed by cardiovascular surgeon Irving Dardik, to study the application of scientific and medical advances to athletics. "We want to develop methods and modalities for working with athletes that would enhance their performances," Dardik stated. As part of this effort, the panel would even "look into areas considered taboo" among members of the public; these would include the possible uses of performance-enhancing drugs.[58] Dardik tried to mollify concerns by asserting at an Athletes Advisory Council meeting that while the "ultimate function . . . of the Olympic Sports Medicine Committee is to provide . . . scientific and technological assistance for maintenance and improvement in athletic performance," the panel would "draw the line where sports medical aid stops and physical manipulation begins."[59] Willye White, who had competed against the East Germans, applauded the USOC plan: "This is the kind of program we've needed for a long time. If the U.S.O.C. lets Dardik operate, there's no telling how far we could go."[60] Most American officials never adopted such a broad interpretation, but Dardik and White's comments are characteristic of the attitude that prevailed within the Olympic movement, which was heavily influenced both by nationalist forces and the increasing popularity of performance-enhancing drugs.

Olympic drug control policies during the 1970s were thus beset by many of the same issues apparent in the previous decade. The various components of the international sport system, including the IOC, its counterparts at the national level, international federations, and organizing committees for the Games, were at odds over both the regulations that should be enacted and how those regulations should be enforced. Nationalistic forces became an especially important component of this environment as countries increasingly perceived the Olympics as a tool for the promotion of their images abroad. The German Democratic Republic, with its extensive doping regime, was the most culpable (and successful) individual country in terms of applying performance-enhancing techniques in the pursuit of this goal. Failing to acknowledge these developments, Olympic policy-makers were slow to take advantage of the latest drug detection methods. As a result, a multitude of athletes, many of whom were unaware as to the substances they were being forced to take, suffered severe—and at times life-threatening—side effects.[61]

The terrorist attacks by the Black September organization at the 1972 Munich Games, in which thirteen Israeli athletes lost their lives, received (quite appropriately) the overwhelming attention of Olympic administrators, media outlets, and government officials.[62] Less justifiable was the relatively anemic response to widespread rumors that East German swimmers were dominating the 1976 Games through their extensive use of performance-enhancing drugs. Although several meaningful changes were made, Olympic officials, still largely approaching the matter through the lens of image management, preferred to downplay the real magnitude of the doping crisis rather than engage in a difficult and expensive process of reform. The IOC leadership continued to favor restricting centralized IOC regulatory responsibility just when nationalistic forces were emerging as a major influence on doping. These forces overwhelmed a vulnerable, internally conflicted policy framework. The stage was thus set for the 1980s, in which a series of doping scandals would finally force the IOC to pursue a new direction.

Five

"IN A FREE SOCIETY,
IT ALL DEPENDS ON US"

In the final decade of the Cold War, the perceived ideological importance of the Olympic movement led to its continuation as a proxy in the political rivalry between the United States and the Soviet Union. At the same time that their respective boycotts of the 1980 Moscow Games and the 1984 Los Angeles Games threatened the future viability of the Olympic movement, the superpowers also had important influences on the direction of doping control policy.[1] Deferring to the wishes of Soviet sport administrators and distracted by the American boycott, IOC leaders failed to fulfill hopes for an effective testing regimen in 1980. As a consequence, the Moscow Games, characterized by de Merode as the "purest" in the history of the movement, produced not a single positive indication of drug use, although unofficial tests later identified a potpourri of performance-enhancing substances.[2] American officials, responding to the athletic successes of the Communist world, weakened their own policies to keep pace in the Olympic medals race. Having largely cast aside idealistic notions that athletics remained uniquely pure in modern society, sports leaders in the United States increasingly perceived these decisions in economic terms. In a quite literal sense, these individuals developed and implemented doping policies with all the cold-blooded skills of a modern corporate executive. The Los Angeles organizing committee for the 1984 Games, motivated by a concern for economic efficiency, exerted particular influence in obstructing expensive testing initiatives.[3] Other members of the international sports community also played critical roles in relaxing doping regulations; at different times during the decade, for example, the IOC medical commission, the International Association of Athletics Federations, and the USOC suppressed test results that would have otherwise rendered athletes ineligible.

While most of the decade was marked by alternating improvements and relapses in regulatory development, the 1988 Seoul Olympic Games, as we will see in chapter 6, served as a turning point in the history of doping control policy.[4] Canadian sprinter Ben Johnson's positive test for the anabolic steroid stanozolol in the wake of a world record–setting 100-meter sprint focused public attention on the issue in a profound way. Government officials initiated investigations into the conduct of the Olympic movement, pressuring Olympic officials to reform their policies. Describing the consequences of these events, IOC member Dick Pound later recalled that "when the definitive history of doping in sport . . . is written, the Ben Johnson disqualification will be one of the key dates. This was a definitive statement by the IOC that it would not cover up cheating, even by one of the leading athletes."[5] Although it would take several years to be implemented, the agenda was thus set for a gradual expansion and consolidation of Olympic drug control policies by the end of the decade.[6]

In the aftermath of a silver medal performance in the 1976 Olympic marathon, U.S runner Frank Shorter was asked whether he planned to compete in the upcoming Moscow Games, scheduled for the summer of 1980. His response highlighted the degree to which performance-enhancing drugs had become necessary to success in elite international sport. "Yeah," he affirmed, as long as "I find some good doctors."[7] The chief American physician at the 1976 Games, John Anderson, predicted "much more of a problem in doping control [in Moscow], particularly in the area of anabolic steroids . . . The majority of the I.O.C. members," he said, "are looking at the trees, not the whole picture." The IOC medical committee was, for example, developing expensive testing equipment while concurrently legalizing known stimulants such as the asthma medication terbutaline. The overly legalistic nature of the IOC's approach ignored the potential of an educational campaign to redirect athletes' moral orientations concerning the use of performance-enhancing substances. Unless rectified, these deficiencies, Anderson argued, were likely to cause a doping catastrophe in Moscow on such a scale as to threaten the future of the movement. "I think in 1980," he concluded, "it will become evident to the world in general and the athlete in particular that man has gone a bit too far in manipulating individuals, and it would seem to this observer that 1984 indeed will come [and go] without the Olympic Games."[8]

Despite such pessimism, several sport administrators believed that a slight retooling of the medical controls would successfully curtail the use of ergogenic aids. Victor Rogozhin, chair of the Moscow Games organizing committee's anti-doping panel, asserted prior to the event's opening that "we have conducted important research on improving methods of detecting steroid hormones and reducing the time necessary for the test. This will make it possible not only to increase the number of tests for this group of drugs, but also to carry them out according to the regulations established . . . by the Medical Commission of the [IOC]."[9] Even American officials expressed optimism; USOC physician Daniel Hanley noted that "the capacity of the labs in Moscow seems to be perfectly adequate, and the testing will be carefully overseen by the Medical Commission."[10]

Meanwhile, athletes and unscrupulous administrators on both sides of the Iron Curtain busied themselves with identifying loopholes in the testing procedures, estimating when they could take the last dose before their competitions. East German scientists implemented a protocol whereby administrations of detectable synthetic anabolic steroids were replaced with injections of Testosterone-Depot and similar compounds in the final weeks before competitions. As "natural" substances, these testosterone doses could not be differentiated through ordinary urinalysis from hormones normally found in the human body.[11] Describing this new "testosterone loophole," an anonymous USOC medical staff member remarked that the "athletes seem to have the timing down to the minute as to how soon they have to 'get off' a drug to avoid detection." A larger infrastructure was, of course, a component of this cat-and-mouse game. "You'd also swear," the staff member continued, "they had Ph.D. pharmacologists working for them to figure out how to beat tests almost faster than the antidoping scientists can make them more sensitive."[12]

Fuel for these suspicions was provided by the revelations of an East German sprinter, Renate Neufeld, who defected and brought along the pills and powders that her coaches had required her to use; chemical analyses later determined they were anabolic steroids. "The trainer told me the pills would make me stronger and faster and that there were no side effects," she explained. Describing the extent of the state-sponsored program, Neufeld declared, "We all lived the same way, the general approach is the same."[13] East German swimmer—and fellow defector—Renate Vogel corroborated Neufeld's account: "You don't know what is being tried out . . . what ingredients there are in the food, what is being injected. You cannot take a stand against it."[14]

In their 1976 proposal, American officials outlined a plan to study the potential of performance-enhancing drugs, but in the run-up to the Moscow Games, they took aggressive measures to combat doping.[15] In November of 1978, a new USOC medical task force recommended the implementation of comprehensive drug tests at all national championships. Describing the proposal as "a positive step," USOC president F. Don Miller asserted that "we have to identify where drugs are being used to centralize our effort. The only way you can do this is through an effective drug testing program."[16] Other Western nations also enacted more rigorous protocols. However, the diffuse structure of the international sport system allowed individual bodies to enact their own preferences, which reduced the likelihood that a global Olympic doping strategy could be created. IOC medical commission member Dr. Arnold Beckett thus complained that "one of the troubles is that there are no totally universal controls. For instance, the United Kingdom and Denmark are quite strict [with doping] . . . But the Soviets will pull their teams out of a competition with testing. And some Americans won't show up, either."[17]

1980 WINTER GAMES IN LAKE PLACID, NEW YORK

Administrators involved in the 1980 Winter Games in Lake Placid, New York, had mixed feelings about the new set of testing procedures planned for the competitions. The costs related to the screens astonished several members of the Lake Placid organizing committee. As head of the committee's marketing department, Norman Hess declared, for instance, that "it would cost Lake Placid far more to provide doping controls than to house and feed the athletes for the whole of the Winter Games."[18] At the same time, however, the doping protocols demonstrated an impressive level of sensitivity. Dr. Robert Dugal, codirector of the competition's doping control effort, asserted that "the system we're using is more sophisticated now. It can separate drugs more precisely and isolate the compounds." His colleague, Dr. Michel Bertrand, went still further: "The equipment acts with the precision of radar," he claimed. "We are confident it will be a deterrent, because athletes who think they can risk trying us will be making a mistake."[19] The head physician for the American team, Anthony Daly, likewise stated that "the old saying was the lab could tell you what kind of lettuce you ate for lunch two days before. Now, I think they could tell you how old the lettuce was. The tests are that sensitive."[20]

Other members of the Olympic medical establishment were less hopeful. Dr. Beckett of the IOC medical commission described the struggle between drug-dependent athletes and doping authorities as "a warfare" in which actions were "ruthless." Asked whether his commission was prevailing, he replied, "No. We can only prevent the more serious aspects of the problem. We win some; we lose some. The war goes on." He perceived a particular danger from the involvement of unscrupulous physicians and sport administrators who either explicitly or implicitly supported the use of ergogenic aids. "Not all the blame should be put on the athletes," Beckett noted. "It goes much further up. The people behind them should be kicked out." As for the integrity of the Games, he asserted that "the competition should be between individual athletes, not doctors and pharmacologists. We don't want sports people used as guinea pigs to boost the doctors behind them."[21] In the end, Beckett's pessimism was validated; the protocols employed at the 1980 Winter Olympic Games in Lake Placid produced not a single positive indication of drug use among the 790 doping tests administered.[22]

The dangerous combination of new doping techniques and political machinations at the Games alarmed several other IOC officials. Having been asked about her perceptions regarding the movement's greatest challenges in the period between the Lake Placid Games and the Moscow Summer Olympics, IOC secretary Monique Berlioux answered that the greatest challenge was "the growing influence of politics in sport and the manipulation of athletes with drugs and the fabrication of an artificial human being."[23] Despite such apparent attention to the problem of doping, the Moscow Games would see no improvement.

1980 MOSCOW OLYMPIC GAMES

In terms of Olympic medical policy, Moscow was a peculiar choice for the Summer Games of the XXII Olympiad because the Soviets were widely believed to have a program similar to that in East Germany. Confirmation of systematic doping by the Soviet Union came in 2003 when Dr. Michael Kalinski, former chair of the sport biochemistry department at the State University of Physical Education and Sport in Kiev, Ukraine, released a 1972 document detailing a clandestine Soviet project in which anabolic steroids were administered to elite athletes.[24] As the 1980 Games neared, however, Soviet sport officials assured the IOC leadership that their regulations would be strictly applied. Indeed, Soviet efforts impressed medical commission chair Alexandre de Merode during an October 1979 tour of the laboratory facilities in Moscow, which he described as "well-equipped."[25] The accuracy of the chair's observations was later called into question, however. Dr. Robert Voy, who became chief medical officer of the USOC in 1984, for example, argued that "after seeing their testing facilities in Moscow firsthand and after realizing the Soviets' willingness to play these types of games, I simply cannot believe that [de Merode's] claim."[26]

Whatever the technological status of the equipment available at the competitions, similar apprehensions concerning the doping preparations in Moscow quickly arose among several observers. The IOC medical commission's Dr. Arnold Beckett expressed some doubt after witnessing firsthand their stunning physiques.[27] Despite these rumblings, not a single competitor failed any of the reported 6,868 gas chromatography tests, 2,493 radioimmunoassay tests, 220 mass spectrometry analyses, and 43 alcohol tests.[28] While most of the IOC leadership basked in the glow of what de Merode called the "purest" Games in the history of the movement, questions remained concerning the integrity of the test results.[29] Manfred Donike, a West German physician on the medical commission, privately conducted his own investigation. Donike had developed a new technique for identifying abnormal levels of testosterone that involved measuring its ratio to epitestosterone in urine (positive tests were set at a 6:1 ratio of the former to the latter). The results of his informal study indicated that the rumors of extensive doping in Moscow had merit. A full 20 percent of the specimens that underwent his testing protocol, including those from sixteen gold medalists, featured testosterone-epitestosterone ratios that, Donike asserted, would have resulted in disciplinary proceedings if the screens had been official.[30]

Thus, these were not the "purest" Games in history; they were likely one of the dirtiest. Athletes did not clean themselves up prior to the competitions—they simply switched to testosterone and other pharmacological agents for which tests remained unavailable. The hypocrisy of the competitions was perhaps best described in a 1989 study by the Australian government: "There is hardly a medal winner at the Moscow Games, certainly not a gold medal winner . . . who is not on one sort of drug or another: usually several kinds. The Moscow Games might as well have been called the Chemists' Games."[31] British journalist Andrew Jennings cited an anonymous KGB colonel as stating that Soviet security officers, posing as IOC anti-doping authorities, deliberately sabotaged the drug tests. Soviets athletes, the colonel professed, "were rescued with [these] tremendous efforts."[32] Whether these claims were true or false, the question was not how the doping policies had succeeded, but why they had failed so miserably. Were the tests deliberately tampered with? Were results suppressed? Could there be a conspiracy? While answers were not forthcoming at the time, future events would provide greater clarity.

In the immediate aftermath of the Moscow Games, the IOC medical commission pushed for more robust doping regulations. De Merode was particularly concerned that the commission's jurisdictional limitation to the Olympic competitions was restraining its success. He pointed out to other IOC members that "it had been hoped to set up some kind of control between the Olympic Games . . . It was essential to continue the work of approving neutral laboratories for doping testing in order that these could be used to test between Games."[33] Dr. Eduardo Hay replied that the politics of the international sport system might make such policy reform difficult. Preaching caution, he stated that "the Medical Commission of the IOC only had jurisdiction within the Olympic Games at present. It would be necessary to modify its role and work with the IFs and NOCs if this authority were to spread to regional Games or international competitions in general." Explaining the nuances of an additional proposal that more athletes should be tested, he continued that "rule changes would create major technical problems," so it was "better to retain the present procedure."[34] For a time, the IOC leadership supported Hay's position.

By May 1982, however, de Merode had made some progress in advocating inter-Games testing. Through negotiations with the international federations, for example, he strengthened an agreement with the International Association of Athletics Federations for procedures through which laboratories could be recognized, and he also established a universal set of sanctions for IAAF track-and-field athletes caught doping between Olympic competitions.[35] In addition, the results of Donike's unofficial testosterone screens in Moscow convinced de Merode that the hormone must be added to the IOC's list of banned substances. In a 1982 interview, he explained that "the increase in testosterone [use] is a direct consequence of the doping control for anabolic steroids. In former times, athletes . . . [had] to stop the use of anabolic steroids at least three weeks before the event. So they have to substitute. And the agent of choice is testosterone—testosterone injections."[36] The IOC soon announced that it was banning the hormone, along with high levels of caffeine.[37]

Not long after the IOC medical commission made this change, there were rumors of a major doping cover-up at the 1983 World Track-and-Field Championships in Helsinki, where the IAAF, rather than the IOC, was in charge of doping control. Given that a number of world records were broken at the event, insiders were convinced of a connection with doping practices. USOC physician Robert Voy specifically pointed to Primo Nebiolo, then president of the IAAF, for the failure to adequately support rigorous protocols. "There is no doubt in my mind," he later wrote, "that, at least in 1983, Nebiolo would not have pressed for honest, accurate testing in Helsinki."[38] Within the IOC leadership, Canadian delegate Dick Pound likewise stated that "something was very, very wrong with the testing procedures [in Helsinki]." He continued, "My feeling was that . . . there either were positives that were not acted upon by the IAAF or that there were directions not to test for certain compounds or substances." Indeed, according to Pound, "all over the world, people shook their heads and said [the testing] is not credible . . . [The IAAF] was in serious jeopardy of becoming a laughingstock because of the results."[39]

A later Canadian investigation revealed that some athletes did in fact test positive for performance-enhancing drugs at the competition. As an indirect consequence of the episode, elite athletes began to appreciate the accuracy of the new gas chromatography and mass spectrometry testosterone tests.[40]

Yet another controversy occurred at the 1983 Pan-American Games, held in Caracas, when twelve members of the U.S. track-and-field squad left before their events to avoid the screens. Several of those who remained were caught and punished.[41] Of greater concern, USOC officials warned several athletes of the more rigorous doping protocols. After learning of the new testing procedures upon her arrival in Caracas, the American team's chief of mission, Evie Dennis, asked U.S. officials to alert their athletes of the screens.[42] "I don't know if anyone of yours is taking drugs," she said to team manager Joe Vigil, "but if anyone is or has, tell him *for God's sake go home.*"[43]

Before the events, a few USOC officials also advocated precompetition tests to prevent unexpected results. Speaking at a July 1983 meeting, USOC member Jack Kelly stated that "one of the things that concerns me a great deal . . . is what would be tremendously embarrassing to the [USOC], and hurt us greatly in future fund-raising, and things of that nature, if several of our athletes were tested for steroids . . . and barred from the Olympic Games." He continued, "I would hope that the Medical Committee would be doing some preliminary testing with the likely athletes . . . to make sure that, when they go to the Games, . . . they are going to pass whatever tests may be used."[44]

USOC president William Simon later admitted that a number of American athletes prior to the 1984 Games failed precompetition steroid screens sponsored by his organization, but were allowed to compete because participation in the testing program was not required.[45] In addition, as only medalists were tested at the Pan-American Games in Venezuela, U.S. weightlifters who failed these preliminary screens, according to Dr. Voy, circumvented the official tests by deliberately performing poorly.[46]

With the 1984 Los Angeles Games looming, American sports administrators and athletes faced dual sources of intense pressure. On the one hand, they were under pressure to demonstrate that they were not doping. Increasingly, doping scandals were perceived as damaging to international sport. On the other hand, U.S. sports officials and athletes were under tremendous pressure to win, especially against the Soviet Union. In the spring prior to the scandal in Caracas, President Ronald Reagan pronounced the Soviet Union an "evil empire" dedicated to world revolution. To win, America needed superiority in all areas of human endeavor. "The struggle now going on for the world will never be decided . . . by armies or military might," the president declared. "The real crisis we face today is a spiritual one; at root, it is a test of moral will and faith."[47]

Reagan framed the Los Angeles Games in terms of these principles. Five days prior to his "evil empire" speech, the president outlined the importance of the competitions to USOC officials:

> Millions of young people will be watching the games as you've been told, young people from all over the world as well as our own children, the fiber of tomorrow's America. And I know we won't let those kids down and won't short-change our country by doing anything less than a first-class job. In a free society, it all depends on us.[48]

Although neither Reagan nor any other member of the U.S. government advocated the use of performance-enhancing substances, such rhetoric made a profound impact on American sports officials. In referencing an aborted blood doping program within his organization, U.S. Cycling Federation official Mike Fraysse rationalized it as a tool for defeating Soviet-bloc teams. "We've been looking into this stuff for years and years and years," he said. "We weren't gonna fall behind the Russians or East Germans any more."[49]

In the early part of the decade, thus, some progress was made in the technical aspects of anti-doping testing, and some steps were taken toward inter-Games testing. An overarching tacit acceptance of doping, however, worked against major progress in anti-doping policy. A primary factor was that East-West rivalry perpetuated the Cold War association between Olympic and political power. The Soviets were reportedly involved in state-sponsored doping, and American leaders, though not directly sponsoring such programs, indirectly contributed to a culture of doping in sports by equating athletic success with national success. And, as we will see in the next chapter, an increasing focus on the financial viability of the Games led to a tendency on the part of some sport officials to view testing as an unnecessary expense. Testing itself was expensive. Moreover, image problems resulting from positive test results, some argued, could undermine financial success—and ultimately, the Games themselves.

Six

TURNING POINT

The USOC continued its policy of testing American athletes in the period before the opening of the Games, conducting testing in the summer of 1984 in the run-up to the Los Angeles Olympics.[1] Drug screens were considered "formal" at the 1984 American Olympic trials in the sense that sanctions were required for positive results, but Dr. Voy later learned that many athletes were allowed to compete despite affirmative indications of doping.[2] In a self-incriminating report that was withheld until after the conclusion of the 1984 Games, USOC president F. Don Miller admitted that eighty-six athletes, including ten at the Olympic trials, had tested positive for banned substances before the competitions in Los Angeles. The timing of this disclosure was, of course, likely motivated by the wish to avert pre-Games criticism of the American team.[3]

The other components of the Olympic governance system, including the IOC and the Los Angeles organizing committee, were motivated less by sincere concerns over doping than by economic issues.[4] The high cost of the 1976 Montreal Games provided a sobering example to officials in California as to the likely outcome of a planning process that failed to incorporate budgetary safeguards. The revenue losses accrued after the U.S.-led boycott of the 1980 Games in Moscow provided additional weight to the lesson. And, in 1980 the IOC elected a new president, Spaniard Juan Antonio Samaranch, who was both more commercially astute than his predecessor and more assertive as a leader.[5] Centralizing decision-making powers within the IOC, Samaranch traveled to over a hundred countries during his first three years as president. In meetings with government officials, he emphasized above all that the Olympic movement should remain insulated from political maneuverings.[6]

The new IOC president combined his political and financial skills with a reluctance to engage with divisive issues. In an otherwise glowing assessment, former IOC marketing director Michael Payne noted that Samaranch's "focus on uniting the Olympic movement meant that, occasionally, he turned a blind eye to indiscretions within the Olympic family."[7] Over time, this tendency posed a significant challenge to those advocating improvements to the existing anti-doping system. According to Pound, the president "always thought the IOC Medical Commission was dangerous" in that its activities might threaten the public image of the movement. Indeed, Samaranch at one point stated, "All they [the members of the medical commission] live for is to find a positive sample."[8]

And in Peter Ueberroth, the Los Angeles organizing committee had a leader with a similar if not greater commitment to economic success. As the former owner of the First Travel Corporation, the industry's second largest in North America, Ueberroth spearheaded an effort that eventually yielded an unprecedented $250 million surplus—the largest in Olympic history.[9] In his memoirs, Ueberroth emphasized that budgetary efficiency proved key to this achievement. "Our mandate," he wrote, "was to stage the Games at no cost to the taxpayer. That was priority number one—to have a surplus, not a deficit. This required fiscal conservatism as well as prudent and responsible management."[10]

Possessing a keen intellect and an assertive managerial style, Ueberroth established a highly centralized organizational structure; other than himself, only a trusted advisor, Harry Usher, possessed any real decision-making authority.[11] Having worked with Ueberroth both in the private sector and on the organizing committee, Patty Patano asserted, "If I had to say Peter Ueberroth equals something it would be control, because his whole life is run on that." Not surprisingly, Ueberroth extended that control to anti-doping arrangements in Los Angeles.[12]

Whether intentionally or not, Ueberroth's focus on the bottom line seemed to influence Olympic policymakers to devote less attention to drug testing. The USOC's refusal to disclose positive drug tests by American athletes prior to the Games, for instance, probably derived from Ueberroth's emphasis on precompetition fund-raising. Revelations about positive test results might have hurt the fund-raising campaign. And, in April 1983, the Los Angeles organizing committee announced that tests for caffeine or testosterone would not be conducted unless the IOC provided convincing proof that the screens were scientifically justifiable.[13] In June, Dr. Anthony Daly, medical director of Olympic Health Services in Los Angeles, outlined the reasons for this position in a letter to de Merode. "We are certain," he wrote, "that the goals of the IOC Medical Commission are precisely the same as those of the LAOOC [Los Angeles Olympic Organizing Committee]—namely, not to permit dope testing which has not been scientifically validated to be performed on athletes during the 1984 Olympic Games."[14]

By November of 1983, Ueberroth had come to believe that the expensive doping regulations constituted a direct threat to the economic integrity of the competitions. He thus wrote to Samaranch that the "drugs and doctors are not only controlling the Games of the XXIIIrd Olympiad, they are beginning to gain control of the whole Olympic movement." In addition, Ueberroth worried about the potentially harmful effects of public disclosures of positive test results. While admitting that "the use of drugs must be curtailed in every way," he asserted that there needed to be a limit. Not only was testing expensive, but disclosures of doping could hurt the Games financially. Implying that economic necessities might trump rigorous adherence to doping regulations in some instances, Ueberroth stipulated that "equally important[,] the dignity of the Olympic movement must be preserved."[15] To undercut anticipated media stories that "all athletes were doped," Ueberroth asked the IOC leadership to emphasize the fact that not all competitors were "drug addicts."[16] The IOC, in Ueberroth's view, should spend less time exposing doping and more time protecting the reputation of its athletes.

In the end, Los Angeles organizing committee members acquiesced to testosterone and caffeine screens after IOC medical authorities affirmed that "these controls were scientifically perfect and not assailable as incorrect."[17] An additional problem arose soon thereafter, however, when athletes were found to be using a lesser-known substance called human growth hormone (hGH) at the 1983 World Track-and-Field Championships.[18] Both scientific and economic hurdles prevented its inclusion on the IOC's list of prohibited substances for the Los Angles Games. The November 1983 medical commission report stated that "a method of detection [for hGH] has been almost perfected . . . but there are very serious doubts as to the real effectiveness of this very costly treatment." The document therefore declared that "it would be premature to draw definitive conclusions and in any case it is out of the question that it be controlled in Los Angeles."[19]

There was also input on doping control at the Los Angeles Games from representatives of Communist-bloc countries. Manfred Ewald, a member of the East German sport establishment, seconded a suggestion by Marat Gramov, chair of the Soviet national Olympic committee, "to carry out doping controls according to politically and geographically balanced viewpoints."[20] Conducting "doping controls in 2 laboratories each in socialist and non-socialist countries," as Gramov proposed in a letter to de Merode, would help "bring about a rather correct and objective doping control."[21]

Soviet-bloc concerns about fairness occurred in the context of heightened hostility between the United States and the Soviet Union during the early and mid-1980s. And, political officials in Moscow were still bitter about the U.S. boycott of the Moscow Games in 1980. Soviet rhetoric thus served in part as a retaliatory mechanism designed to embarrass the United States. Some evidence suggests, however, that Gramov's statements reflected a fear within the Soviet Union that their country had fallen behind the United States in the Olympic medals race. From the perspective of policymakers in Moscow attuned to international perceptions of geopolitical power, the prospect of a poor performance in Los Angeles seemed dreadful—especially when contemplated alongside Soviet military failures then taking place in Afghanistan.

Nevertheless, the prospect of defeat at the hands of Americans appeared less ominous than other possibilities that might ensue in Los Angeles. If a U.S. victory on its home territory frightened Soviet leaders, the risk that the GDR might surpass the USSR in Olympic success appeared downright cataclysmic. Under the laws of Soviet geopolitical physics, a satellite allowed to spin out of control threatened the integrity of the entire imperial system. Whether resulting from concerns over testing protocols or from the dangers posed by East German doping, fear of failure reinforced the arguments in favor of a boycott. Remembering the mediocre Soviet showing at the 1984 Winter Games in Sarajevo, Ueberroth certainly believed that visions of failure affected Soviet policymakers. In outlining several factors for the boycott decision, he stated:

> I believe completely without question that before Sarajevo, the week before, the day before, all systems were go for their competing in the Games . . . [However,] they didn't do well, and this is way underestimated in the eyes of the West. And they were severely criticized at home because they didn't perform well. The East Germans beat them in the measurements that count, the amount of gold medals and the premiere sports and the projections that they went there with. And remember this, they had sold their public in 1980 that their eighty gold medals truly reflected their Summer Games power, and that the few countries that didn't come there were not significant in terms of medal winning.[22]

American competitors shared this assessment. Track-and-field superstar Carl Lewis later recalled that "most of their [the Soviets'] athletic programs were in a period of transition. They were conducting a lot of new experiments, and I just don't think they were ready."[23]

In addition to concerns raised by Eastern-bloc countries, a number of IOC members from several Western nations were apprehensive that U.S. judges might interfere if and when American athletes were detected using performance-enhancing substances. At a July 1984 meeting, Italian delegate Franco Carraro accordingly asked de Merode to provide "assurance that the doping tests in Los Angeles would be held under strict conditions." Although de Merode recognized that "if an American athlete had a test that was positive, the IOC might be taken to Court," he told Carraro that "this consideration should not prevent the IOC from doing its work."[24] In his pre-Games official report, de Merode downplayed the issue by emphasizing the positive steps that had been taken in Los Angeles. "The laboratory is perfectly equipped," de Merode declared. With respected physician Don Catlin as its director, he continued, the laboratory "has acquired remarkable experience and is perfectly satisfactory." As for the earlier tension between the IOC and the Los Angeles organizing committee regarding the testosterone and caffeine screens, de Merode stated that all difficulties had been resolved.[25] The drug tests, including testosterone and caffeine screens, would be "objective, firm and comprehensive, and any positive cases would be dealt with in accordance with IOC Rules."[26]

De Merode's initial hopes for a set of rigorously enforced doping protocols in Los Angeles went largely unfulfilled, however. U.S. athletes won a spectacular eighty-three gold, sixty-one silver, and thirty bronze medals—and not a single American was included on the list of those found to have been doping.[27] Indeed, the fact that only twelve Olympians tested positive for performance-enhancing drugs suggests that the IOC's doping control efforts had made little progress since the 1960s. The absence of positive drug screens was perhaps due less to Olympic doping policies than to the destruction of test results before they could be disclosed to the public. Before the opening of the Games, the Los Angeles organizing committee had refused to provide IOC doping authorities with a safe. This resulted in the theft of a number of medical records at the competitions. With few exceptions, the consequent lack of evidence made sanctions impossible.[28]

While some suspected that de Merode played a role in the scheme, others, recalling Ueberroth's hostility toward rigorous tests, placed the blame squarely on the shoulders of local authorities.[29] In a 1994 letter, de Merode claimed that the organizing committee's Dr. Tony Daly at first explained that the documents had been shipped to IOC headquarters in Switzerland, but then, after further questioning, admitted that the papers had in fact been destroyed.[30] Describing his frustration over the episode, IOC member Dick Pound later wrote that the disappearance of documents "led to the perception that the IOC was soft on drugs and that it did not want to find positive cases at the Games, but it was the L.A. organizing committee that had removed the evidence before it could be acted on by the IOC."[31]

Local officials, of course, denied any complicity. The associate director of the laboratory handling the tests, Dr. Craig Kammerer, stated that "we were totally puzzled initially and figured that something must be going on, politically or a cover up."[32] As a self-described "cynical idealist," Pound did not absolve the IOC leadership from all responsibility.[33] According to Pound, IOC president Samaranch conspired with his IAAF counterpart, Primo Nebiolo, to delay the announcement of a positive test result to make sure that the competitions in Los Angeles ended without significant controversy.[34] Elaborating on their possible motives, medical commission member Dr. Arnold Beckett asserted that "it would have done quite a lot of damage if five or six . . . of the positives . . . had led to the medal winners . . . Some of the federations and IOC are happy to show that they're doing something in getting some positives, but they don't want too many because that would damage the image of the Games." As a result, Beckett elaborated, "We [the IOC medical commission] took the responsibility of not revealing [the destruction of the documents] publicly."[35] Image and commercial viability were of primary importance in the Samaranch presidency, even if at the expense of regulatory responsibility and integrity.[36]

LEGACY OF THE LOS ANGELES GAMES

Several new forms of doping in Los Angeles highlighted the dynamic nature of the drug problem. Athletes were by now adept at finding alternative performance-enhancing techniques by the time a new drug screen was developed. At the 1984 Games, five medal-winning U.S. cyclists received blood transfusions prior to their races from prominent cardiologist Herman Falsetti.[37] The idea of autologous blood transfusion was to preserve an athlete's red blood cells and then introduce them into his or her body immediately prior to a competition. Because red blood cells carry oxygen, the reintroduction of a half-liter of blood provides the human organism with a roughly equivalent amount of oxygen per minute.[38] Although the practice is now known as "blood doping," the procedure did not violate IOC regulations in place at the time. As Thomas Dickson, the team physician who witnessed the transfusions, put it, "They were certainly unethical, [but] whether they were illegal is something I still don't know."[39]

Whatever the moral dimensions of the episode, the United States Cycling Federation (USCF), as the national governing body for the sport, split the difference between apathy and responsiveness. While an apology to the American public was issued and the officials involved in administering the transfusions were punished, federation president David Prouty announced that "no athletes will be held or considered responsible." Describing the cyclists as unsuspecting victims, he asserted that "nothing should be considered to have tainted any medal" won by them.[40] Seeking a more active position, USOC executive director F. Don Miller wished to supplement the IOC's antiquated rules with policies promulgated by his own organization. Speaking at a February 1985 USOC meeting, he argued that "it has not been declared illegal in the past by the IOC medical commission, simply because . . . there was no medical tests [sic] for blood doping, and that almost invalidates our whole system of laws." Miller proposed that the USOC executive board take the position that "blood doping is, in fact, a form of doping, and is illegal." After all, he concluded, "there are other methods of proving that people have broken the law."[41] U.S. government officials also took notice. Citing public health concerns—several of the cyclists who received transfusions in Los Angeles became ill—National Institutes of Health official Dr. Harvey Klein urged Olympic administrators to prohibit blood doping at their competitions.[42]

By this time, the IOC was taking notice, too. Swedish delegate Matts Carlgren told his counterparts at a December 1984 IOC session that he "believed that the main problem concerning the future of the Olympic Games was not participation but doping." Proposing more funds for medical research, he argued that "the IOC ought to lead in this domain and analyse the threats drugs impose [on] sport."[43] Several months after Miller's criticism of the IOC's lax position toward performance-enhancing blood transfusions, de Merode announced that his commission had decided to ban the practice. "Although no feasible detection test is available at the present time," he stated, "the Commission feels that it is a question of ethics."[44] Describing the difficult negotiation process through which the policy was promulgated, de Merode stated that "with this aim in mind, the Commission . . . met with representatives from the IAAF, the AIBA, the FINA and the IWF." Enforcement of the rule, according to de Merode, would be no less complicated: "Steps should be taken, in collaboration with the IFs," he concluded, "for the standardisation of methods and procedures of the laboratories."[45]

Unofficial tests in Los Angeles also indicated that a majority of the athletes competing in the pentathlon had used beta-blockers during the event.[46] Indeed, before the Games, the IOC medical commission had expressly permitted their dispensation for "therapeutic" purposes upon presentation of certificates issued by athletes' personal physicians.[47] By reducing blood pressure, heart rate, and blood vessel constriction, these drugs, normally used to treat hypertension and heart disease, steadied the hands of pentathletes during the shooting components of their competitions.[48] While nothing could be done about the situation in California, de Merode declared the following year that the administration of beta-blockers for the purpose of enhancing performance would be considered, like blood doping, an illegitimate practice.[49]

The blood doping scandal in Los Angeles served as a focusing event for the USOC. In March 1985, the organization announced a comprehensive plan calling for rigorous drug screens at all major events in the period before the opening of the 1988 Olympics in Seoul. In terms of punitive measures, the proposal included an escalating set of punishments; first offenses would result in a one-year suspension while second offenses would result in a four-year suspension, which would preclude participation in Seoul. "Wherever the athletes compete," said USOC director of sports medicine Kenneth Clark, "they'll be tapped on the shoulder and told it's time for the urine sample." While the USOC leadership was eager to accept the plan, the support of the national federations that governed individual sports was less certain. To his credit, USCF president David Prouty announced that the suggestion was "terrific" and that "philosophically, it meshes perfectly with what we want to accomplish."[50] By June 1985, however, the plan, which would go into effect at that month's National Sports Festival in Baton Rouge, had been changed to meet the approval of the national federations.[51] Although the USOC committed $800,000 to a comprehensive testing regime, the enforcement mechanisms were significantly weakened. Rather than an escalating set of punishments controlled by the USOC, athletes would be sanctioned only at the behest of the national governing bodies of their respective sports.[52]

These modest steps did little to improve the situation in the four years before the next Olympic Games. Nationalist forces again played a part in weakening doping regulations in international sport at the 1986 Goodwill Games in Moscow. The U.S. team traveling to Russia was told that all competitors would be subjected to rigorous drug inspections after their events.

The Americans reportedly ceased their anabolic steroid cycles well before the competitions. "What they found in Moscow, however," Dr. Voy later wrote, "was something quite unexpected. There wasn't any drug testing." Apparently, the U.S. squad was deliberately "burned" in order to foster the notion that the Communist bloc, despite its absence in Los Angeles, still reined supreme in elite international athletics.[53] While such machinations may have had perceived short-term political benefits, many Soviet athletes, like those in East Germany, were afflicted with subsequent medical problems. Prior to the 1984 Games, an unofficial study cited the widespread administration of performance-enhancing drugs to Soviet athletes as the primary reason for their high mortality rate, which had been accelerating since the mid-1970s.[54] The actions by Soviet administrators at the 1986 Goodwill Games demonstrated that the report had had little effect in moderating their policies.

Many of the national governing bodies and international federations that governed individual sports were equally reluctant to toughen their enforcement of doping regulations. In 1987, both the IAAF and its American counterpart at the national level, The Athletics Congress (TAC), managed to circumvent positive test results. At that year's National Outdoor Championships in San Jose, TAC officials avoided a finding of guilt for American discus champion John Powell by citing minor procedural errors in the labeling of his "A" and "B" specimens by Dr. Harmon Brown, head of the organization's medical committee.[55] Later that year, the IAAF weakened its testing system at the World Track-and-Field Championships in Rome by replacing IOC doping physicians Manfred Donike and Arnold Beckett with several less qualified individuals.[56] Demonstrating how far unscrupulous members of the elite sports establishment would go to avoid detection, Charlie Francis, then coach of Canadian sprinter Ben Johnson, told a colleague at the event that his protégé had gonorrhea to rationalize the presence of the steroid-masking agent probenecid (which could be justifiably used as an adjunct in treating the disease) in his system.[57]

Still, Samaranch was confident enough to claim in January 1987, "You may rest assured that we shall be very firm where doping is concerned . . . It is a form of cheating which we cannot tolerate."[58] At the 1988 Winter Olympics in Calgary, he continued this theme. "Above all," he stated, "such behavior makes a mockery of the very essence of sport, the soul of what we, like our predecessors, consider sacrosanct ideals." Samaranch thus resolved, "Doping is alien to our philosophy, to our rules of conduct. We shall never tolerate it."[59] The IOC, however, did not live up to Samaranch's lofty words in the run-up to the 1988 Games. De Merode later admitted destroying a list of names of fifty-five athletes who had been detected doping in the six months prior to the opening of the 1988 Games in Seoul.[60] Given de Merode's long tenure trying to make the anti-doping effort better, this action perhaps reflected a temporary moment of panic—albeit one that would in the long run undermine his credibility.

CRISIS: THE 1988 SEOUL OLYMPIC GAMES

Johnson's positive test for probenecid foreshadowed deeper troubles for the Canadian sprinter and the Olympic movement. On September 24, 1988, Johnson defeated American track star Carl Lewis in the 100-meter sprint, lowering his previous world record to 9.79 seconds. Two days later, Francis, "about 42 hours after my life's greatest moment," was awakened by a knock on his door from Dave Lyon, manager of Canada's track-and-field squad. "We've got to get over to the Medical Commission," Lyon said. "Ben's tested positive [for steroids]." As Francis realized, a positive test for a major athlete was serious business: "The track federations had staged drug tests for 20 years," he later wrote, "and in all that time no major star had failed one—not officially, at any rate."[61] Upon being told that there was "terrible" news, Dick Pound asked IOC president Samaranch, "Has someone died?" Samaranch replied, "Is worse [sic] . . . Ben Johnson . . . has tested positive."[62] Although the sprinter initially claimed that someone might have spiked his urine after the race, the IOC quickly found Johnson guilty and stripped him of his medal.

Public reaction was swift, as various observers set about predicting the consequences of the event. In the aftermath of the race, American sprinter Edwin Moses anticipated that "this will change the history of the Olympics . . . This will change a lot of people's lives."[63] Johnson's own financial losses were catastrophic. After the race, the sprinter's manager, Larry Heidebrecht, asserted that "the total endorsement power that he has following the world record and gold medal would certainly put him into seven figures . . . How many millions, I wouldn't want to speculate."[64] The economic juggernaut came to a sudden stop after officials acknowledged the test results to the public. The Italian sportswear company Diadora, mirroring the actions of several other enterprises, immediately canceled its five-year, $2.4 million contract with the runner, and the Japan-based Kyodo Oil Company terminated a marketing campaign featuring Johnson.[65] Estimating the financial loss for the sprinter, Heidebrecht later stated that the scandal cost Johnson

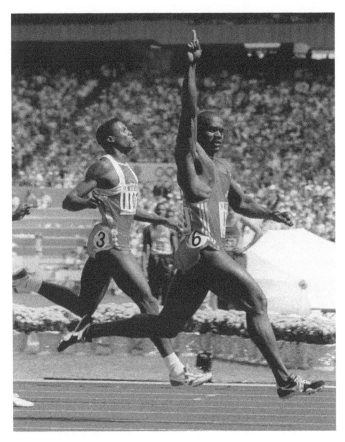

FIGURE 5.   *Seoul, Democratic People's Republic of Korea: Ben Johnson (right) of Canada crosses the finish line to win the Olympic 100-meter final for a world record 9.79 seconds at the Olympic stadium, September 24, 1988. Johnson was later disqualified for failing to pass a drug test (ROMEO GACAD/AFP/Getty Images).*

a staggering $25 million in endorsement deals.[66] Johnson, as put by Canadian IOC member James Worrall, had thus "just been killed as an athlete, and probably his complete life has been ruined."[67]

Other occurrences concerning the competition also demonstrated the dynamic nature of the doping problem. Soviet leader Mikhail Gorbachev himself ordered that all Soviet competitors had to pass precompetition drug screens. Coaches and administrators who failed to ensure this result would receive serious punishment, Gorbachev warned.[68] According to a 1989 issue of the Soviet publication *Zmena*, a $2.5 million laboratory aboard a vessel sailing off the Korean coast had provided precompetition screening to Soviet competitors. Due to fears that instances of doping would be revealed, several athletes, according to the report, were not allowed to compete.[69]

In addition, Bulgaria and Hungary both pulled their weightlifting teams from the Games after several of their athletes tested positive for performance-enhancing substances.[70] Both in the 1988 Olympic trials and at the Games themselves, U.S. officials barely escaped disqualification of several athletes. At the trials, eight track-and-field athletes were found to be using the prohibited substance ephedrine. Using a loophole in U.S. rules whereby athletes were provided a one-time "inadvertent use" defense in the case of a positive test at a national competition, U.S. officials were able to escape punishment. Then, during the Games, a member of a prominent American team was found to have an abnormally high testosterone level, which should have resulted in the disqualification of the entire squad. U.S. officials, however, convinced the IOC that the athlete's normal production of the hormone was elevated.[71]

IOC officials optimistically portrayed these incidents as doping policy successes.[72] Taking the positive view that Johnson's test would catalyze future anti-doping efforts, Dick Pound proclaimed that "this is a disaster for Ben, a disaster for the Games, and a disaster for track and field. But let's turn this around to make the slate clean and show the world that we do mean business. We are prepared to act." Better attuned to the public perception of the Olympic movement, President Samaranch was downright cheerful in an interview: "We are showing that the system works," he declared. "We are showing that my words are not only words, they are facts. We are winning the battle against doping."[73] Experts in the field, however, presented evidence to the contrary. After the Games, USOC chief medical officer Dr. Robert Voy estimated, for instance, that over 50 percent of those competing in Seoul had used some form of performance-enhancing substance.[74]

THE INTERNATIONAL POLITICS OF DOPING AT DECADE'S END

In addition to embarrassing Olympic administrators, the events in Seoul galvanized government officials in the home countries of banned athletes. The Canadian national government appointed Charles W. Dubin, associate chief justice of the supreme court of Ontario, as chair of a special commission charged with investigating drugs in athletics.[75] After nearly ten months of public hearings broadcast live on Canada's TSN network and 14,817 pages of testimony from 119 witnesses, Dubin issued his report.[76] Arguing that Olympic doping policies were overly narrow, he wrote that while "the athletes who cheat must, of course, bear their full share of responsibility . . . the responsibility cannot be solely theirs."[77] The report continued, "Until now, the focus has been only on the athletes. It is obvious that a broader net of responsibility will need to be cast. Coaches, physicians, therapists, and others involved in the care and training of athletes cannot escape responsibility for the sorry state of sport today."[78] In the wake of Johnson's test, several IOC officials expressed similar beliefs. Canadian IOC member James Worrall declared, for instance, that "obviously, people behind . . . [Johnson] are responsible . . . Ben is a lad who will follow instructions. If he is told that something is good, he will believe it."[79]

Exacerbating the problems caused by such unscrupulous individuals were organizational conflicts within the Olympic governance structure that prevented the promulgation and enforcement of a universal set of doping regulations. Describing the diffuse nature of this system, Dubin noted that the collective "failure of many sport-governing bodies to treat the drug problem more seriously and to take more effective means to detect and deter the use of such drugs has . . . contributed in large measure to the extensive use of drugs by athletes."[80] Similarly, Dick Pound asserted that Johnson was "a pawn in this, the host organization for the substance." The sprinter's use of steroids, Worrall stated, "points up the tragedy of the whole system."[81] Both the Canadian special commission and members of the IOC, then, conceived the doping problem as systemic and asserted the need for a wider range of enforcement mechanisms.

While setting the agenda in terms of this policy development was relatively simple, actually accomplishing a coordinated approach to doping was far more complicated. The first step in this process had actually occurred before the Seoul Games, in late June 1988, at the first World Conference on Doping in Sport, chaired by de Merode and attended by delegates from twenty-six countries. The conference yielded the proposal of an anti-doping charter to be signed by both private sports authorities and national governments.[82] At the Seoul Games, de Merode announced the formation of a new working group composed of international sports authorities that would be "responsible for working out this strategy so that it is adhered to by all sporting nationals at a governmental level, and by all international authorities."[83] Samaranch echoed this emphasis on coordinating the anti-doping effort in a November 1988 speech in Moscow. "In order to overcome the scourge of doping," the IOC president asserted, "all our forces must be united and a concerted effort made by sports and civil authorities working together in perfect harmony."[84]

Several developments in the Soviet bloc also provided a catalyst to policy change. First, increasing numbers of Soviet athletes were leaving the country for lucrative contracts in Western Europe, hurting the country's competitiveness at elite events.[85] Second, several satellite countries in Eastern Europe began during the 1980s to assert their independence through sport.[86] Third, the relative political openness produced under Glasnost led a few sports officials to confirm the reality of doping in Soviet sport. For example, after the Seoul Games, senior Soviet track-and-field coach Igor Ter-Ovanesyan asserted the need for greater state involvement on the issue. "I think," he said, "that society needs proper legislation to combat this evil, seriously punishing both doctors and athletes, coaches and drug suppliers."[87] Finally, policymakers in Moscow realized that their scientists could not keep pace with Western pharmaceutical advances in terms of the development of new performance-enhancing substances. Consequent to these developments, Soviet sports authorities took a position of leadership in pushing for the implementation of de Merode's universal system of doping control.

At a November 1988 UNESCO (United Nations Educational, Scientific and Cultural Organization) meeting held in Moscow, sports leaders from 100 countries signed a statement of support for the IOC's proposed antidoping charter. Although there was no enforcement device, IOC official Alain Coupat declared that "this is a big day for the I.O.C. . . . . It means UNESCO recognizes that the fight against doping must be constructed on a global basis, not by state, and that the I.O.C. is the best organization to direct the fight."[88] Since the United States did not belong to UNESCO, Soviet officials came to a separate, preliminary agreement with American leaders that would allow their respective doping experts to test each other's athletes.[89] This cooperative arrangement was later expanded to include Great Britain, Australia, West Germany, Sweden, South Korea, Italy, Norway, Bulgaria, and Czechoslovakia.[90]

From the perspective of broader international developments, it should be noted that Moscow's efforts on the issue occurred alongside an ambitious rethinking of Soviet power in the world. Believing that the Soviet Union could no longer act out of self-interest alone, Gorbachev wished to strengthen Moscow's role in international institutions. During a December 1988 speech before the United Nations, he declared:

In the past, differences often served as a factor in pulling away from one another. Now they are being given the opportunity to be a factor in mutual enrichment and attraction. Behind differences in social structure, in the way of life, and in the preference for certain values, stand interests. There is no getting away from that, but neither is there any getting away from the need to find a balance of interests within an international framework, which has become a condition for survival and progress.[91]

At the IOC summer 1989 general session, de Merode advocated the creation of a new doping commission within the IOC. Composed of IOC medical commission members as well as representatives from national Olympic committees and international federations, the new commission, he stated, would meet every year to consider how positive tests should be addressed. The commission would be supplemented with an IOC-run "mobile laboratory" that would enable a program of out-of-competition testing to begin.[92] De Merode envisioned that the IOC would remain in command of the new anti-doping commission, but as it turned out, an independent anti-doping organization would be founded in November 1999.

The 1980s saw a series of crises that collectively led to a paradigm shift in Olympic doping policy. In the early years of the decade, most policymakers believed that the doping issue was of secondary importance to the 1980 and 1984 boycotts. At the same time, Olympic leaders such as IOC president Samaranch and Los Angeles Olympic organizing committee head Ueberroth took the stance that the IOC medical commission was overzealous and that the reputations of Olympic athletes needed to be safeguarded from potentially damaging scandal. This conceptualization of the doping problem led to a belief that the problem could be best addressed by either obscuring its true extent or by actively suppressing instances of doping. And, as in the 1960s and 1970s, this culture of denial was exacerbated by the loose system of Olympic governance, through which a variety of organizations could set their own degrees of compliance with doping regulations.[93] The respective cover-ups at the 1983 World Track-and-Field Championships and Pan-American Games by the IAAF and the USOC were direct results of this regulatory framework. The IOC, though more progressive than national committees and international federations in terms of doping, also engaged in questionable behavior; uncertainties remain, for instance, as to the degree of Samaranch and de Merode's complicity in destroying test results at the 1984 Los Angeles Games.

In the end, these activities set the stage for the single most important event in the history of Olympic doping policy: the disqualification of Ben Johnson at the 1988 Games in Seoul. As Dick Pound noted in 1989, "There have been positive tests and disqualifications on other occasions, but never one which has attracted such scrutiny and created such concern."[94] At last convinced as to the necessity of state intervention, the deeply embarrassed Canadian government called attention to the inadequacies of the existing system. The Soviet Union, having suffered a diminution in global status and having concluded that it could not keep pace with Western pharmacological advances, also insisted on comprehensive reform. Although a universal doping authority would not come into existence for almost another decade, a political climate conducive to its creation now existed.

Seven

TOWARD A
            UNIFIED APPROACH

The dismantling of the Berlin Wall, which began in November 1989, signaled the end of the GDR sport machine and revealed the secrets of its extensive doping system.[1] The subsequent collapse of the Soviet empire likewise resulted in broadened prospects for a more cohesive political process regarding the doping issue. In Asia, a rise in indications of doping among athletes from the People's Republic of China was met with official prohibitions against performance-enhancing substances in that country.

Although organizational hurdles remained, leaders in both governmental and nongovernmental bodies engaged in efforts to merge the powers of the existing set of doping authorities.[2] Over the course of the decade, this process included a series of international conferences that collectively led to the creation of the World Anti-Doping Agency (WADA) in November 1999. Through the involvement of the United Nations, multiple national governments, and leading private sports organizations, the agency was given a more aggressive mandate to both promulgate and enforce doping regulations within the Olympic movement.[3]

Because the IOC "embargoes" its internal publications and memoranda for a period of twenty years, it is difficult to discern the actual deliberations of IOC leaders during the 1990s. However, the available evidence suggests that the IOC's avoidance of moral leadership remained relatively unchanged during the decade. Thus, while there was progress during the 1990s toward the development of a universal regulatory system, principally due to the threat of governmental involvement, the decade was also characterized by the same unscrupulous practices and questionable regulatory judgments that had weakened previous initiatives. As the turn of the decade approached, IOC vice president Dick Pound acknowledged in July 1989 that the movement's understanding of the doping problem had developed little since the 1960s, asserting, "We still have no clearly stated definition of what doping is."[4]

In addition, President Samaranch failed to effectively guide the IOC on doping policy throughout the rest of his tenure. Samaranch was primarily concerned with the economic vitality of the Olympic movement. As de Merode stated, "Samaranch knew he needed money to develop the IOC, that without it we were beaten, but the problem with money is that you are under the influence of it."[5] Worried that his movement was beginning to suffer financially from adverse publicity regarding its increasing number of drug scandals, Samaranch attempted to undermine the established belief that doping constituted an ethical crisis. In July 1998, for example, he asserted that policies based on philosophical notions of "fair play" were excessive in that "for me, everything that does not injure the health of the athlete is not doping."[6]

At the same time, bodies such as the Court of Arbitration for Sport, created in 1983 as an alternative to public judicial venues, often undermined doping decisions by the IOC leadership. These influences, although fostering significant short-term obstacles to a coordinated approach, over the long term forced Olympic leaders to develop a more professional set of regulations. The restructured governance system did, in the end, play an important role in constructing the broad political support needed for the long-term success of WADA.

In the January 1990 issue of the IOC's *Olympic Review,* President Samaranch outlined several anticipated developments in the post–Cold War international sports environment. Averring that the end of the superpower conflict was in part due to the internationalist ideology of the Olympics, he declared that "the unity of our Movement is triumphant. This unity has opened up perspectives, freed an undreamt-of development potential that would have been unthinkable only ten years ago. Our task is now to turn these promises into action." The events of the previous few years, Samaranch continued, also held important implications for the battle against performance-enhancing drugs. Envisioning a peace dividend of transnational cooperation, he sought to reverse skepticism regarding the IOC's previous inaction, stating, "The fight is now being waged daily, and all, whether athletes or those around them who look after them, must be aware of their own involvement, and seek to combat all cheating and misconduct."[7] In this regard, Samaranch's administration presented several new ideas as means to go beyond the limited on-site drug screens that were at the traditional center of Olympic doping policy.

For future out-of-competition examinations, which most knowledgeable observers believed necessary for effective regulation, Olympic officials proposed a mobile, flying laboratory to extend the temporal and geographic reach of their tests.[8] De Merode stated that "these anti-doping measures, and those taken by other sports organizations and government bodies, could have an impact on the results of the [1992 Olympic] competitions in Barcelona."[9] Such a step toward out-of-competition testing was in fact long overdue. Speaking at a 1991 international conference on sport law, Robert Armstrong, an attorney who had worked on the Canadian investigation after the Ben Johnson scandal, asserted that "the IOC and its Medical Commission have known for years that testing for anabolic steroids at the competition was a virtual waste of time in terms of providing effective deterrent for their use during training periods."[10] Although encouraged by the potential of the mobile laboratory, Samaranch nevertheless noted that to ward off future criticism, "much still remains to be done towards standardizing the application of sanctions in the event of a positive test." Again commenting on the possibilities afforded by larger global developments, he emphasized "how vitally important it is for us to define and implement, without haste yet also without false modesty, a sports policy which is adapted to the new political, social and economic circumstances of our planet."[11]

Despite such statements, the Olympic doping-control system remained organizationally and politically fragmented; it was, as a consequence, largely ineffectual at the beginning of the decade. The Court of Arbitration for Sport (CAS) constituted an additional factor in the already diffuse regulatory framework.[12] At first, the CAS allowed IOC leaders to more easily keep doping controversies from the public eye by preempting public judicial proceedings. According to committee member Anita DeFrantz, Olympic leaders saw this as the primary function of the court. "The intention," she noted, "was to keep sports matters out of ordinary courts."[13] For the first decade of its existence, the CAS functioned perfectly on this point. "The IOC had considerable control of the organization," DeFrantz continued, "and was able to amend its statutes and rules."[14]

Over time, however, the body's decisions began to dilute the ability of the IOC to avoid unwanted interference on the issue. In a 1986 advisory opinion concerning the possibility of a lifetime ban for individuals caught using performance-enhancing substances, the CAS pronounced, for instance, that every action by an international sport body—including the IOC—must conform to basic principles of fairness; only *deliberate* offenses against legitimately promulgated and enforced rules and procedures would therefore warrant such a far-reaching punishment.[15] While useful—and perhaps even necessary—for the protection of athletes' rights, such decrees provided significant obstacles to the type of tough countermeasures that many believed were needed by the IOC. In the longer run, though, these activities obliged Olympic policymakers to promulgate more rigorous standards for their own conduct; only a threat to its power could induce the IOC to take such substantive action.[16]

Because a more rigorous approach had not yet been developed, though, national sport bodies continued to dampen transnational anti-doping activities. In contesting charges of anabolic steroid use at an August 1990 track-and-field meet in Sweden, 1988 U.S. silver medalist Randy Barnes—the reigning world record holder in the shot put—filed an appeal alleging "erroneous doping procedures" after he tested positive. Because the test occurred at an overseas competition, the case was reviewed by the International Association of Athletics Federations, which served as the international federation for track-and-field. The IAAF recommended a two-year suspension. Rather than confronting the IAAF, Barnes used his status as an American competitor to petition The Athletics Congress (TAC), the sport's governing body in the United States, to overturn the IAAF ruling against him.[17] A similar TAC appeal by U.S. sprinter Butch Reynolds, who had received a silver medal at the Seoul Games, likewise highlighted the problem of overlapping jurisdictions on doping questions.[18] These episodes also suggested that American sport bodies were falling behind their international counterparts in terms of their reputation for fairness on drug issues.

While one three-member TAC panel eventually—and quite surprisingly—supported Barnes's punishment, another panel ruled that Reynolds was innocent of the IAAF's charges. Dr. David Black, testifying as an expert witness, first called into question the validity of the data derived from the drug screen that was employed. Then, Reynolds's legal team demonstrated that the seal on the container in which the sprinter's urine had been stored could be "picked," thus successfully challenging the "chain of custody" of the sample.[19] The sprinter's two-year suspension by the IAAF was accordingly lifted within the context of domestic competitions, although the IAAF's punishment could not be challenged at the international level. Elaborating on the contradictory effects of this outcome, Greg LaShutka, who served as Reynolds's attorney, commented that "now we're on a collision course between TAC's executive director [Ollan Cassell] and the IAAF."[20] The lack of clarity regarding organizational authority again undermined effective regulation.

In spite of the IAAF ruling against Reynolds's participation in international competition, the sprinter remained optimistic that he would be allowed to compete in the forthcoming Barcelona Games, scheduled for the summer of 1992. In October 1991, Reynolds stated that "right now, I'm in the Olympic trials, and I hope that once I earn the right to represent the United States at the Olympics, I will be able to go to the Olympics."[21] The TAC's reputation for duplicity concerning the issue did little to persuade Reynolds's fellow competitors of its integrity.[22] After its decision to restore the sprinter's domestic eligibility was announced, British track star Linford Christie lamented that "the state of the sport at the moment is disgraceful." Christie (who was himself later convicted of doping), continued, "Sometimes, I'm just embarrassed to be among these people and I'm glad I'm near the end of my career and not starting it. He [Reynolds] is going to retire a very rich man while the rest of us are still running our legs off."[23] The episode also demonstrated that conflicts among anti-doping agencies would continue to allow utilization of performance-enhancing drugs to go unpunished.

Reynolds, who stood to lose millions of dollars if the international ban continued, eventually sought and won an injunction against the IAAF.[24] A U.S. district judge awarded Reynolds $27.3 million in damages.[25] Upset by the prospect of significant economic losses in the future, IOC leaders vowed to rework their strategies. In what had become a predictable pattern, a circumstance that threatened the profitability of the movement once again catalyzed action by Olympic leaders who would otherwise have preferred more restraint. De Merode, as head of the IOC medical commission, stated that "we are making a review of all our procedures and regulations . . . We are sure we will be in a position where it will be impossible to find any failure in these rules."[26]

For its part, the IAAF deemed the award "worthless" due to a belief that the U.S. court lacked jurisdiction over IAAF measures.[27] And, although the award was eventually reversed, the case did much to convince Olympic leaders of the need for a central mechanism through which a more coordinated regulatory strategy could be promulgated; judicial proceedings involving the Olympics entailed costly attorney's fees, judicial awards, and damage to the movement's already tarnished image.[28] Obscuring the underlying motivations for this position, de Merode shrewdly claimed that public courts—as opposed to IOC officials like himself—"are not interested in knowing if somebody has taken some banned drug but only in finding any kind of mistake in the procedure."[29]

THE IOC DEALS WITH
EAST GERMAN DOPING

In addition to administering performance-enhancing drugs to thousands of East German athletes, GDR officials took steps to ensure that their doping program would remain a secret. Information concerning East Germany's doping regime began to surface after the disintegration of the country in November 1989, however. Late the following year, the German magazine *Stern* published a report on the activities of a former GDR doping center near the Bavarian town of Kreischa. The facility, according to the article, provided precompetition tests to ensure that no East German athlete would be caught using performance-enhancing substances outside the country's borders. Six individuals, including three gold medalists, were specifically named as participants in the program.[30] A pair of German researchers, Dr. Werner Franke and Brigitte Berendonk, later added substance to these allegations by appropriating a documentary collection of East German Stasi reports and doctoral theses written by scientists participating in the program.[31] In 1991, the preliminary findings of this husband-and-wife team were published in Berendonk's groundbreaking book *Doping Dokumente.*[32]

Rather than viewing the East German scandal as a legitimate ethical concern, however, Olympic officials once again approached the issue as one requiring image management; actual punishments for those involved in the GDR doping system were therefore not initially considered. In elaborating the official IOC position, de Merode declared that "what we are dealing with here is a certain kind of public relations issue. The public must be persuaded that something is being done." For him, this required little substantive response in that the IOC need only provide "moral credit" to the work of others.[33]

And, realizing that a stable German presence was essential to the financial future of the Olympic movement, Samaranch focused on the steps required for a unified German team and expressed enthusiasm for a possible bid by the city of Berlin to host the 2000 or 2004 Olympic Games.[34] Upon visiting former East German sports leaders shortly before the publication of *Doping Dokumente,* he downplayed their culpability, stating that "damage to the high performance sports of the G.D.R. would be not only a damage for Germany but also for [the] whole Olympic movement."[35] As for the possibility of punitive steps, the IOC president opposed the administration of ex post facto penalties; in January 1998 he stated, "There are time limits, one cannot go back that far."[36] The basis for Samaranch's position was economic in nature: "We now have a more critical situation than ever," he said, "with revelations of systematic drug-taking by competitors in Germany over the years . . . This could be seriously damaging financially, with the loss of sponsorship."[37]

TENTATIVE STEPS TOWARD A GLOBAL STRATEGY

Despite the IOC's indifference, the growing number of drug allegations persuaded Olympic officials that the public had to be convinced that effective policies were being developed to prevent future problems. In a July 1991 speech at the opening of the IOC general session, Samaranch pronounced that "doping is cheating, and is in absolute contradiction to the Olympic ideals of fair play and loyalty." Expressing a profound—if historically dubious—dedication to the eradication of prohibited performance-enhancing activities, the IOC president assured his audience that "the IOC has fought against this scourge not only with words but also, and especially, with effective measures." Nevertheless, more should be done, according to the president. "For this," Samaranch stated, "we would like all International Sports Federations to adopt the same measures against drug abuse."[38] Efforts for the harmonization of Olympic doping policies were thus given a new rhetorical emphasis.

The Third Permanent World Conference on Anti-Doping in Sport, held a few months later, provided the next forum for discussing the process of unifying drug policies; topics included long-term plans for "international-cooperation and co-ordination" of doping regulations.[39] Athletes in attendance expressed a surprising level of commitment to the rigorous sanctions proposed for those caught using prohibited ergogenic aids. Peter Radford of the British Sports Council presented survey findings that 24 percent of the athletes in his country supported five-year suspensions for those who failed drug tests; even more astonishing, 51 percent agreed with the imposition of lifetime bans in certain instances. Radford, perhaps conscious of the IOC leaders in attendance, remarked, "Elite athletes . . . would not be as squeamish as officials in dealing out harsh punishment to their drug-taking colleagues."[40]

In addition to ideas for tougher penalties, several delegates suggested that a broad-based educational campaign would provide an effective complement to this more punitive anti-doping system. "The emphasis will have to be placed on educating the athletes about the health hazards of anabolic steroids," said Paul Dupre, president of Athletics Canada, "and I believe it's only then we will be able to overcome this problem."[41]

Testing, of course, was a central topic of concern; testing techniques were fraught with challenges. Inadequacies in the urine tests then in use by Olympic authorities led the IOC medical commission to consider more sensitive blood screens that could identify prohibited substances.[42] The growing use of "blood doping" with the hormone erythropoietin (EPO) was a particularly important catalyst for such tests in that EPO could not ordinarily be detected in an athlete's urine. De Merode's refusal to consult the other bodies in the Olympic governance structure before bringing the proposal before the IOC executive board provoked significant interorganizational conflict, however. As a result, the suggestion failed to receive the political support necessary for its immediate implementation.[43] Individual miscalculation coupled with political fragmentation undermined a potentially useful new policy. De Merode nevertheless suggested that his organization's anti-doping efforts were beginning to succeed. He reported that 61,000 drug screens were conducted in 1991, representing a 36 percent increase from the previous year; more importantly, out-of-competition tests had increased by 92 percent. These activities, according to the medical commission chair, collectively resulted in a net 1 percent drop in positive drug tests for the year in Olympic sports.[44] (De Merode failed to show any link, though, between the higher number of drug screens and the lower percentage of positive tests; athletes might have simply discovered other loopholes in the IOC's drug protocols.) In any event, due to these perceived successes, out-of-competition screens were the focus of de Merode's future testing prescriptions. In September 1991, a temporary IOC commission for such testing was created, with de Merode stating, "This is an area where there really is work to be done."[45]

Despite de Merode's public display of optimism, other doping experts remained unconvinced that a significant turning point had been reached in the struggle against performance-enhancing drugs. Dr. Donald Catlin, a member of the IOC medical commission and head of doping control at the 1984 Los Angeles Games, believed that while the use of illicit ergogenic substances might have been decreasing in the Western nations, it was proliferating in several areas of Eastern Europe that were still coping with the end of the Cold War. "Worldwide," he declared in July 1992, "I feel we're making real progress . . . But we can't pretend the problem is over." Catlin continued, "Clearly, in some countries, there is still a lot of work to do. In some areas, we have no doping controls at all."[46] Beliefs that pharmaceutical advances in richer countries allowed them an advantage remained wide-spread among the former members of the Soviet bloc. Looking back on his time in office, long-serving Bulgarian weightlifting coach and official Norair Nurikian later asserted:

> Athletes [in Bulgaria] take some stimulants, but because we are lagging well behind the advances in medicine . . . well, there are many cutting edge drugs that are very clean but those cost hundred times more. So, because we are falling behind we use some dated things while the technologies are highly advanced and keep advancing. With all due respect . . . take the American athletes for example. How would they be able to run so incredibly—with scotch and lemonade? No way![47]

The newly unified Germany was by then experiencing intrastate tensions due to the fallout from the public exposure of the GDR doping system. In the winter of 1992, a media frenzy ensued when three former East German athletes, including 100-meter world champion Katrin Krabbe, were found substituting another person's "untainted" urine for their own while training in South Africa.[48] The trio's controversial coach, Thomas Springstein, complained about the polarizing effects of such allegations, stating, "I have no good relations with any western coaches . . . They do their work, I'll do mine. There's lots of talk about east-west togetherness on the team, but there's been very little success." As for disparities within the squad as a result of the matter, he stated that "our athletes are sent to doping tests at every turn, while the western athletes hardly ever get checked." Springstein was not alone in his criticisms. "What impertinence!" German Olympian Sigrun Grau lamented. "Our western colleagues accuse east athletes of doping with no proof. I can only hope we will be a real team in Barcelona."[49]

In addition to highlighting the challenges caused by the formation of a new global environment, the episode demonstrated the problems still inherent in international sport's doping regulatory system. Springstein's employment was terminated and the three runners received four-year suspensions by the German national track-and-field federation, but the athletes cited flaws in the testing procedures in their appeals of the decision.[50] Because the German federation had requested its South African counterpart to conduct the actual urine collections, questions arose as to the propriety of the arrangement. Dutch attorney Emil Vrijman, acting on behalf of the athletes, asserted that the "[IOC] charter for doping in sports says very

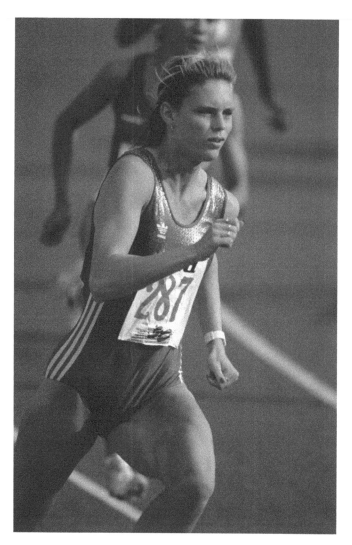

FIGURE 6.   *Katrin Krabbe of East Germany, winner of the women's 200-meter*
final, at the fifteenth European Athletics Championships, held in
Split, Yugoslavia, in August 1990 (Bob Thomas/Bob Thomas Sports
Photography/Getty Images).

clearly that in order to have your athletes tested abroad, you should have
an agreement [on testing procedures] between federations." In this case,
he continued, "the Germans didn't know how the South Africans tested
. . . No procedural guidelines were drawn up."[51] Such concerns were later
given credence when Sam Ramsay, South Africa's leading Olympic official,

criticized the anti-doping effort on his continent as "a relatively lackadaisical one."[52]

Ramsay's statement did not directly influence the case, as it was made several months after the decision, but under mounting pressure, the German federation reduced Krabbe's ban from four years to one; this, in turn, angered IAAF officials. Calling the decision "absolutely ridiculous," IAAF staff member Enrico Jacomini argued that "there is no such thing as a one-year ban. If she's innocent, there's no ban. If she's guilty, she serves four years."[53] Taking control of the case, the IAAF circumvented the problems caused by the procedural inconsistencies in South Africa by invoking a regulation allowing two-year suspensions for those who bring "disrepute" to the sport of track-and-field.[54] Although her running career was effectively terminated, Krabbe sought recourse in the German judicial system. In 1995, a Munich-based regional court ordered the German track-and-field federation and the IAAF to pay the runner $2.7 million in lost wages, stating that they were "not competent" to impose such a sanction.[55] As in the past, the divided policy environment through which such issues were addressed undermined the effective enforcement of anti-doping regulations.

At the 1992 Summer Games in Barcelona, cracks in the Olympic regulatory structure remained apparent. Although medalists were automatically tested in most events, only two of the top four finishers in swimming were screened for drugs. As a result, Chinese swimmer Zhuang Yong did not undergo examination after winning the women's 100-meter freestyle competition. "I think that all gold medalists should be drug-tested," complained U.S. swimmer Jenny Thompson, who was tested after finishing behind Yong. "They do it random here," she explained, "and I wouldn't mind, if I got a gold medal, getting drug-tested."[56]

Further, there were still varying understandings about banned substances. British sports officials were frustrated when several of their athletes—initially cleared following testimony by Olympic doping expert Arnold Beckett—were asked to leave Barcelona after drug screens revealed the pharmacological agent Clenbuterol in their systems. Beckett, it turned out, thought the substance was permitted; other IOC members believed that although the substance was not specifically listed, it fell within the IOC's prohibited class of substances related to anabolic steroids.[57]

Outside the private sports system, political leaders focused on establishing a stronger governmental anti-doping presence in terms of both legislative power and oversight mechanisms. An item placed on the agenda of a 1991 UNESCO conference in Paris thus contemplated the potential utility of a binding intergovernmental legal instrument.[58] A UNESCO study issued the following year as to the feasibility of such a mechanism asserted that the longstanding absence of national and international governmental bodies in the existing anti-doping framework should be reconsidered:

> National and international legal instruments are few and far between. They are to be found mainly within the regional European framework and are not effective enough to be feared . . . Furthermore, the only instrument of international scope, the International Olympic Charter against Doping, does not emanate from a governmental organization. It has coercive effects only within the amateur sports movement, the maximum penalty being exclusion from the sports federation or from the Olympic movement and a ban on practicing the sport in question within that federation.[59]

The expensive legal proceedings of the previous year nevertheless reinforced the existing skepticism among international sports leaders as to the desirability of additional governmental involvement. Believing instead that public courts should be avoided at all cost, these officials agreed in the summer of 1993 on the implementation of a universal set of doping principles to be enforced by a new, private arbitration system with a more robust CAS as its nucleus. In addition to suggesting that international and national federations adopt the IOC's list of banned substances, these bodies were asked under the agreement to join a multilateral enforcement system. To avoid troublesome public judicial proceedings, athletes, under the agreement, would be required to submit their disputes to a "Supreme Council of International Sport Arbitration" before being allowed to compete. "The decisions of the arbitration tribunal will be equivalent to the final decision of an ordinary civil appeals court," stated IOC director general François Carrard, in reference to the tribunal's membership of twenty international jurists and a set of expert arbitrators. As for the combined effects of this arrangement, de Merode optimistically declared that "I would say this is a historic step . . . We have followed up words with real action."[60]

Despite the rhetoric, the autonomy of the CAS would remain conjectural until recognized by public judicial institutions. Happily for those wishing to undercut increased governmental influence, the uncertainty ended in 1994, when the Swiss Federal Tribunal rejected an appeal of a CAS decision and confirmed the organization's autonomous jurisdiction over disputes in international athletics.[61]

Olympic doping policy thus remained in flux during the early 1990s. With Cold War tensions over, former members of the Soviet bloc no longer sponsored national doping programs; for their part, Western governments no longer turned a blind eye to performance enhancement on their own national teams. Indeed, national political units became the primary catalysts of reform. The restructuring of Olympic doping policy was slow, however. Most Olympic officials remained wedded to the notion that national political involvement should be avoided rather than welcomed. The partnership that would eventually form between private and public authorities at the end of the decade was by no means assured. It would require the continuing engagement of national authorities as well as greater flexibility on the part of the IOC leadership.

Eight   CHALLENGE AND
PARTNERSHIP

From the perspective of global political affairs, the opening to the West of the People's Republic of China during the 1970s and 1980s proved transformative. After nearly three decades of absence, the PRC rejoined Olympic competition at the 1980 Winter Games in Lake Placid, New York. As the contacts between the PRC and the outside world grew over the following decade, PRC scientists gained increasing access to Western pharmaceutical information, and Chinese athletes soon began to employ doping techniques at elite competitions.[1]

The conclusion of the Cold War exerted a profound influence over the way in which foreign audiences perceived these developments. After 1991, many American and European observers identified the PRC as the heir of their former Soviet enemy. A number of Western athletes competing at the 1992 Barcelona Games believed that the PRC operated a state-sponsored doping regime similar to the one conducted by East Germany prior to the end of the Cold War. Some even claimed that there were suspicious links between Chinese sports officials and former GDR coaches. Seeking to dispel these rumors after Chinese swimmer Lin Li set a new world record in the 200-meter individual medley, coach Zhang Xiong asserted that while "an East German coach came to China in 1986 . . . [Lin Li] has never trained with East German coaches."[2]

When three runners from the PRC swept the women's 3,000-meter race at the 1993 World Track-and-Field Championships in Stuttgart, a frustrated Canadian competitor, Angela Chalmers, remarked that Chinese doping was "pretty obvious, in my opinion." Believing that PRC scientists were taking advantage of loopholes in IAAF drug regulations, she asked, "What can we do? They don't fail the tests." For Chalmers's coach, Doug Clement, the discrepancy between Chinese male and female performances was telling. "When you see that pattern," he asserted, "where the women suddenly go ahead and the men don't make such a huge impact, there is a concern that the response to anabolic agents would be much bigger in women than men."[3]

At the conclusion of the competitions in Stuttgart, a grassroots campaign for a crackdown on Chinese doping developed among Western journalists, athletes, and sports officials.[4] "Something has to be done," argued Chalmers. "We've witnessed some things that are pretty scary." Fellow Canadian runner Leah Pells likewise alleged that "it's very strange that a couple of years ago they were nowhere to be seen in any middle distance events for women—heats, finals, anywhere . . . And now they're winning literally everything." Perhaps remembering the complicity of East German public officials, Chalmers asserted that their Chinese equivalents should be the prime targets of any future investigation. Stating that "I feel really sad for the athletes more than anything," she emphasized her belief—which corresponded with that of many others—that "it's a [doping] system."[5]

Despite increasingly vociferous calls for a response, Olympic leaders were reluctant to act aggressively. Having been informed that seven Chinese swimmers failed drug tests between 1991 and 1993, for example, the IOC refused to take action.[6] Following positive indications of drug use by eleven Chinese swimmers at the 1994 Asian Games in Hiroshima, de Merode personally discounted the possibility of officially sanctioned Chinese doping, stating instead that the results were nothing more than "accidents that could happen anywhere."[7] Diverting responsibility from his organization, IOC director general François Carrard argued that "Chinese sports authorities are doing their utmost to control the doping problem."[8] Why the IOC chose not to respond was predictably left unstated.

Leaders in the PRC initially blamed racist sport officials in Japan (a traditional rival of China) for manufacturing the test results; only slowly did they acknowledge Chinese culpability. Even then, government officials refused to acknowledge any sort of state-sponsored program, instead blaming individual coaches and athletes.[9] Nevertheless, the PRC's announcement—however reluctant—that it would initiate an investigation of the events in Hiroshima again demonstrated the heightened interest on the part of national governments in the aftermath of the Ben Johnson affair.

A lukewarm response from the International Swimming Federation (FINA) failed, however, to satisfy observers hoping for a crackdown on Chinese transgressors. At the conclusion of a 1995 joint visit by FINA and Olympic Council of Asia officials to Beijing, the organizations together announced that the controversy was "purely individual cases which cannot be generalized for other athletes who have performed and shown their talents and abilities in all fairness."[10] Indeed, according to the announcement, there was "no evidence that the Chinese are systematically doping athletes."[11]

Aware that more Chinese medals meant fewer for their own athletes, national organizations of other countries reacted far more aggressively. The German swimming federation, for example, bypassed IOC officials, who it believed were inadequately addressing the situation, declaring that it would boycott the forthcoming World Cup in Beijing. "We do not want to be a part of an event that is a doping nest," explained German federation official Ralf Beckman.[12] Australian swimming officials were even more assertive, insisting that the PRC doping regime dictated a four-year ban of Chinese swimmers from international meets.[13] As a charter member of the Pan Pacific Swimming Association, Australia also voted with American, Canadian, and Japanese administrators against Chinese participation in their organization's 1995 championship meet.[14] Elaborating on the reasons for the decision, Carol Zaleski, president of the U.S. swimming federation, said the decision meant that the "Chinese know the world is looking at them, and we're not going to let the history of East Germany repeat itself."[15]

In the wake of such calls—and to the amazement of many in the West—Chinese officials enacted a series of domestic reforms. The Communist *People's Daily* published a new anti-doping policy in March 1995. In addition to proclaiming an official prohibition on performance-enhancing substances, the text declared that coaches and athletes would thenceforth be subjected to lengthy suspensions for breaches of anti-doping rules; sports administrators and physicians involved with doping would also face significant penalties. Soon thereafter, the Standing Committee of the National People's Congress promulgated a National Sports Law to add substance to this approach.[16] For a time, the policy seemed to work. At the 1996 Olympic Games in Atlanta, not a single athlete from the PRC failed a drug test; and Chinese swimmers captured only a single gold medal.[17] Notably, IOC officials had virtually no hand in these positive steps; they were the work of national political authorities.

1996 ATLANTA GAMES

The 1996 Atlanta Games sparked an increase in the level of commitment by American sports officials to the fight against doping. With the United States hosting the competitions, even the highest levels of the American government expressed interest in the matter, perhaps in the hope of preventing embarrassment. Attending an IOC executive board meeting approximately a year prior to the competitions, U.S. vice president Al Gore remarked that the founding philosophy of the Olympic movement included respect for "a healthy body and a healthy mind. It means athletes who are drug free." Praising the IOC's efforts to combat drugs, he noted that "there is more we can do" in terms of providing educational and psychological support to athletes. As for refining the code of penalties for those caught cheating, Gore stated that "it may also be time to apply the same strict penalties—if not more serious ones—to coaches, trainers, and administrators who know of, and therefore condone, drug use."[18] While falling short of proclaiming official federal involvement, Gore's enthusiasm nonetheless set the agenda for a greater commitment to anti-doping by private U.S. sports bodies.

In April 1996, the USOC passed a code of conduct for its athletes and revised its out-of-competition testing protocols, which provided forty-eight hours prior notice to athletes before drug screens could be conducted. USOC president LeRoy Walker stated, "We have to do what is required. We used to worry about an athlete smoking a cigarette or drinking a 3.2 beer. We've gone beyond that."[19] Similarly, USOC executive director Dick Schultz declared that "we want to set the standard for the world." The USOC program nevertheless had several defects—it would cost $2.8 million a year and would not be fully implemented until after the Atlanta Games were concluded.[20]

The latter point was made somewhat less disappointing when the testing program for the competitions in Atlanta was announced. Indeed, the facilities and personnel to be used were more extensive than for any previous Olympic competition; at a total cost of $2 million, 600 medical staff members would conduct an anticipated 1,800 drug screens using several new, highly sensitive mass spectrometers. The chief medical officer in Atlanta, Dr. John Cantwell, who described the anti-doping task as "the equivalent of eight Super Bowls a day for 17 days," accordingly predicted a four-fold increase in the number of athletes found using anabolic steroids compared to the number caught at the 1992 Games.[21] USOC vice president Dr. Ralph Hale was far less optimistic. "Our anti-doping campaign," he lamented, "has been a failure to this point. Many countries have lost confidence in our anti-doping effort. I'm not sure we're doing the right job."[22] Several potential methods of detecting human growth hormone could not be finalized in time for their implementation in Atlanta.[23]

The prospect of a higher number of drug disqualifications due to the IOC's enhanced testing instruments worried several U.S. sports leaders. As head of the U.S. track-and-field federation, Ollan Cassell warned that "to introduce something that's questionable, which hasn't been proven and there's so few of these in the world, the IOC is taking a big chance."[24] De Merode, believing that legal issues constrained the committee's ability to impose penalties, declared that the screens would be allowed only for the purpose of "further study." Consequently, the IOC fell short of fully supporting this component of the Atlanta Games testing program. The integrity of the Olympic movement was again subjected to public question after facts concerning the episode were released.[25]

More important from the perspective of political sovereignty, the U.S. government surrendered its jurisdiction regarding disputes at the competitions to the CAS. Outlining the need for this agreement under new CAS procedures designed to accelerate the resolution of disputes, IOC member Anita DeFrantz later wrote, "This required an understanding with the U.S. judiciary, both state and federal, that the CAS had jurisdiction over these cases and that only in cases where due process was not made available could the national courts become involved."[26]

This, however, reflected only a narrow retraction of governmental involvement. USOC leaders began in the aftermath of the competitions to collaborate with American government officials to realize the USOC's newly ambitious anti-doping effort. In late 1997, committee president Bill Hybl sent a letter to FBI director Louis Freeh requesting the investigation of a suspicious internet website claiming to offer illicit performance-enhancing substances. Asking the bureau to "pursue all avenues to determine if this kind of Internet advertising can, by any legal means," be obstructed, Hybl stated that the USOC was "committed to ensuring a level playing field for all athletes, and this kind of advertising has the potential to destroy the careers and health of existing and aspiring Olympians alike."[27] For their part, USOC officials subsequently proclaimed that random, out-of-competition drug screens would begin at each of their training centers.[28]

THE FINAL PUSH FOR UNIFICATION

At the same time, a convoluted set of judicial proceedings was again demonstrating the problems caused by the lack of a unified regulatory system, bringing into question the legitimacy of both national and international doping decisions. When fifteen-year-old American swimmer Jessica Foschi was put on probation and then given a two-year suspension by the U.S. swimming federation after she failed a 1995 steroid screen, her family filed suit in a New York state court, alleging that the organization had misconstrued its own regulations.[29] U.S. swimming federation president Carol Zaleski argued that the suspension was mandatory: "We are bound by the rules of our international federation . . . It's clear that a two-year sanction is what is required under the FINA rules."[30]

Further complicating matters, the U.S. swimming federation, under threat of Foschi's lawsuit, later rescinded its decision, leaving the question of a possible suspension to FINA officials.[31] Foschi then successfully convinced an American Arbitration Association panel, operating under the charter of the USOC, to remove her probationary status.[32] Angry at the interference of American judicial bodies, FINA eventually reinstituted the two-year suspension at the international level.[33] Controversy at the 1996 Olympic Games was averted when Foschi failed to qualify for the U.S. team, but the organizational confusion of anti-doping policy continued. The Court of Arbitration for Sport reduced FINA's suspension to six months, which was itself backdated to the day of the failed test.[34]

In a controversial decision at the Atlanta Games, organizational factionalism was again demonstrated when the CAS declared that the IOC had inappropriately included bromantan, a stimulant manufactured in Russia, on its list of prohibited substances.[35] The IOC disqualifications of five athletes from the former Soviet bloc who tested positive for the substance were accordingly reversed. Explaining the decisions, CAS general secretary Jean-Philippe Rochat stated, "The experts were not totally sure that bromantan was simply used for the sole purpose of enhancing performance."[36] The IOC leadership, however, saw the episode as a blatant usurpation of its authority. IOC vice president Dick Pound, for instance, later asserted that by adding to the public disaffection that had begun with the Ben Johnson scandal, the CAS pronouncement "simply reinforced the idea that the IOC talked a lot but did nothing to ensure that its own Games were clean."[37]

Similar disputes in other countries led several international athletic federations to rewrite the punitive clauses of their own regulations. The IAAF, for example, was confronted by a growing number of challenges in Asia and Europe on the basis that its longstanding policy of four-year bans for certain doping violations infringed upon athletes' rights to work. The IAAF accordingly announced that the rule "cannot be enforced in a number of countries due to conflicting national legislation." Because national federations could choose to keep the suspensions under their own codes, an inequitable regulatory system developed under which athletes from some countries faced much harsher penalties than those in others.[38] On a broader level, the IOC effectively conceded that its plans for a universal anti-doping approach had failed. "There is not yet a satisfactory definition of doping," lamented IOC director general François Carrard. For him, the agenda for the forthcoming September 1997 IOC general session was clear: "simplify, unify and become more effective."[39]

Believing likewise that the existing IOC medical code was, as demonstrated by the CAS decisions, "impossible for anyone to enforce properly," Pound noted that "once the final decisions moved from the IOC Medical Commission to an independent arbiter, the IOC might well find itself without a legal basis for its actions, such as disqualification of its athletes."[40] President Samaranch only made matters worse by proclaiming that the IOC's list of banned substances should be reduced by making legal everything not detrimental to the health of an athlete.[41] This apparent attempt to abdicate moral authority over doping issues was, as Pound later recounted, "like pouring gasoline on a fire that was already burning."[42]

Within the fracturing IOC leadership, de Merode implicitly criticized Samaranch by commenting that "the people who want to reduce the list are the people who want to let doping function."[43] After Samaranch rescinded his controversial statement, IOC authorities addressed the problem by focusing upon the creation of a new anti-doping code. It became apparent that this was another half-measure, and Pound suggested at an emergency 1998 meeting of the IOC executive board that there was a need for an independent authority to spearhead the battle against performance-enhancing substances.[44] "This agency will make us stronger than before," de Merode argued after the meeting. "To be united is a key success of the anti-doping fight. We all have to be unified in this battle."[45]

Even then, the chances for the implementation of a different approach would have been negligible in the absence of governmental pressure developing out of two additional scandals. First, French police discovered a smorgasbord of banned substances during a raid on hotel rooms occupied by competitors in the 1998 Tour de France. Later that year, the U.S. Justice Department began an investigation connected to allegations of bribery in the IOC's decision to award the 2002 Winter Games to Salt Lake City.[46] Having avoided public law enforcement mechanisms for decades, the IOC leadership was shocked into a new openness regarding governmental involvement in doping regulation. Better to establish a partnership with public bodies now, IOC leaders reasoned, rather than risk a complete takeover at some point in the future.[47]

The World Conference on Doping in Sport, to be held in February 1999, consequently received the support of the Olympic leadership. Anita DeFrantz later noted:

The negative publicity of the various scandals combined with the realization among leaders of the Olympic Movement that national law enforcement officials were beginning to take the lead in doping control through raids on sport teams and other means prompted the IOC to convene the World Conference on Doping in Sport.[48]

Samaranch, by now attuned to the possibility of a cataclysmic scandal, wrote that the conference was conceived "so that all the parties concerned can reflect and make a firmer commitment to the fight against doping, which is poisoning the world of sport. We have won several battles, but we have not yet won the war."[49] De Merode, meanwhile, hoping to lessen the prospects of expensive legal proceedings, proposed that punitive measures be reduced for those caught using banned substances. Catalyzing widespread condemnation, this suggestion again sparked the interest of national governments. U.S. deputy drug czar Donald Vereen, for instance, responded to the medical commission chair that "we are troubled that such a compromise could be seen as undermining the strength of purpose with which the IOC is determined to tackle the drug use and doping problem." Vereen continued, "It may create . . . a widespread perception that [the] conference lacks the ability and wherewithal to adopt the types of strong changes needed to address the problem."[50]

In light of the considerable legal, political, ethical, and financial difficulties that would attend the development of a coordinated approach, the IOC extended conference invitations to the United Nations and a number of national governments.[51] As a result of the meeting, the "Lausanne Declaration" was adopted by the delegates, which called for the institution of a number of interconnected measures. The most important of these was the notion of a new anti-doping authority, which the IOC promised to support with an initial allocation of $25 million.[52]

Samaranch initially envisioned this agency as operating within the IOC—and thus remaining under his control.[53] This idea, however, failed to satisfy government authorities. British sports minister Tony Banks emphasized that "the chairing of the independent agency by President Samaranch would compromise it and that is something we would not be happy to accept."[54] Barry McCaffrey, then director of the U.S. Office of National Drug Control Policy, agreed: "The I.O.C. is rushing forward to build an institution that we cannot support—one that is more public relations ploy than policy solution."[55] Given the widespread skepticism regarding the in-

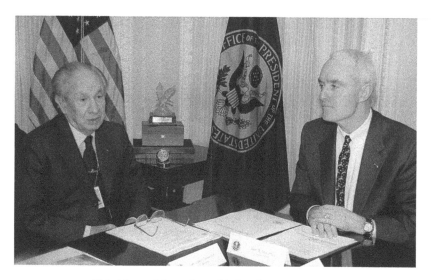

FIGURE 7.   *U.S. National Drug Control Policy director Barry McCaffrey (right)*
and IOC president Juan Antonio Samaranch discuss the process of
improving the World Anti-Doping Agency during meetings on Decem-
ber 14, 1999, in Washington, DC (MARIO TAMA/AFP/Getty Images).

tegrity of international sports leaders, governmental officials such as Banks
and McCaffrey enjoyed considerable leverage.

Understanding the power dynamics of the organizational debate, Pound
sought to make the best of the IOC's relatively weak bargaining position.
Rather than insist on maintaining absolute control over doping policy, he
argued that the committee should seek to maximize the benefits of a con-
cession. He thus reasoned to Samaranch:

> We already know that the Olympic movement is incapable of
> controlling the use of drugs in sport on its own. We do not
> have the legal or the financial means to do so and, frankly,
> there is little enthusiasm for the struggle itself among many of
> the IFs . . . [Alternatively,] if we bring the governments to the
> table as full partners we will have all the necessary means at
> our disposal, and we can lay off half the costs of the initiative
> on them.[56]

Although at first reluctant to forfeit administrative authority over doping matters, Samaranch eventually agreed to a hybrid public/private organizational model. Under the plan, private and public authorities would

share equally in both decision-making power and financial responsibility.[57] In light of Banks's and others' wishes, private sports leaders were pleased that private authorities would still have a significant part in regulation.[58] In the final analysis, then, a narrow yielding of power to an anti-doping body functioning under shared responsibility appeared tolerable—especially when measured against the alternative outcome of even greater government control.

The World Anti-Doping Agency started its work in November 1999 with the ambitious aim of becoming fully operational by the 2000 Summer Games in Sydney.[59] With Pound as its inaugural president, the agency held its first board meeting on January 13, 2000, during which an agenda was established for the intermediate future.[60] Speaking at that meeting, Pound expressed his hopes for a revolutionary system that could challenge the ongoing proliferation of performance-enhancing activities in elite-level athletics. Pound declared:

> Neither the public nor the sports authorities could bring about a complete solution to the problem of doping in sport alone; they had to work together with a common objective to achieve what no one had achieved to date. WADA was an independent agency which had to demonstrate by its actions and commitment that it was worthy of public confidence and of the athletes whose integrity it was charged with protecting.

With these notions in mind, Pound optimistically predicted that "13th January 2000 would be looked backed [sic] upon as an important date in sport history."[61] Developments in the next century of Olympic competition would determine whether these remarks were valid.

The 1988 Ben Johnson scandal and the end of the Cold War both had a profound impact on Olympic anti-doping policy. Media reports and the attendant public outcry were coupled with increasingly forceful government voices. National political bodies pushed sports organizations throughout the 1990s to institute a new approach toward doping. Despite these pressures, Olympic officials remained reluctant to impose substantive reforms. In the end, however, a continuing set of public scandals, ranging from the exposure of the GDR doping system to the Salt Lake City bribery episode, captured their attention. And, while their actions were slow to bear demonstrable results, Olympic officials did engage in a process that eventually led to a collaborative anti-doping framework. The series of international conferences through which leaders in both the public and private sectors conferred was particularly important in refashioning political perspectives away from a longstanding ambivalence toward drugs in elite athletics. In producing the type of policy environment necessary for the creation of WADA in late 1999, this framework demonstrated a newfound commitment to multilateral activities that had been absent in previous undertakings.

The new anti-doping agency faced many challenges. Chief among these was the consolidation of control required for the type of robust activities envisioned by its founders. Given the natural propensity of individual organizations to maintain power whenever possible, several of the units in the Olympic governance structure were reluctant to surrender their influence over doping policy. At the same time, WADA scientists were faced with a multitude of new performance-enhancing substances and techniques. Indeed, the specter of such possibilities as gene manipulation threatened to undermine existing beliefs that the battle against doping could actually be won.[62]

Nine A NEW CENTURY

$\mathbf{A}$s IOC president Samaranch approached retirement in the summer of 2001, he was hopeful about the continued financial viability of the Games, but he expressed pessimism about the battle against doping: "in doping, you can only get partial victories."[1] The Olympics were reaching record levels of financial success, as exemplified by the IOC's successful negotiation of a set of contracts collectively worth $1.3 billion for the broadcast rights of the 2000 Sydney Games. At the same time, however, a variety of new performance-enhancing techniques were coming into use.[2]

Presenting fresh challenges to Olympic officials, several of these practices, including the revolutionary possibilities of gene manipulation, could not yet be detected. "As if all the 'regular' doping were not bad enough," lamented Dick Pound in 2006, "we are about to see genetically modified athletes. I have no doubt that genetic manipulation experiments are already underway to improve sport performance."[3] Fortunately for policymakers in the movement, the decades-long process of power consolidation over doping regulation that culminated in the creation of WADA allowed resources to be quickly redirected toward scientific matters.

The new agency itself benefited from the continuing commitment of public authorities to the eradication of prohibited ergogenic aids in elite international athletics. This support was best expressed by a 2000 study partially funded by the U.S. Office of National Drug Control Policy. The report stressed the societal importance of sport. "Because of the mutually reinforcing relationships among sports, the family, education, the economy, politics and religion, the impact and reach of sports in our society cannot be overstated," the report stated.[4] Addressing the negative influence of the still fragmented Olympic governance system, the study posited, "The crazy quilt of jurisdictions responsible for anti-doping policies and practices . . . assure[s] inconsistency in applying any rules."[5] While the creation of WADA in November 1999 constituted a promising development, WADA could thus far only make "recommendations" to the IOC. It was therefore necessary to "ensure that an independent international organization [WADA] exists with authority over the methods of measurement and sanctions for doping in Olympic sports."[6]

The inaugural meeting of the WADA foundation board, held on January 13, 2000, in Lausanne, was well attended. Hopes were high that WADA, supported by both public and private funds, would have the requisite degree of autonomy to eliminate doping in high-performance sport. Failure, noted Denis Coderre, Canadian secretary of state for amateur sport, "could be the end of the Olympics."[7] The meeting's impressive list of participants included four physicians, several attorneys, a university professor, and nine individuals with prior government experience. In welcoming them, Pound, the body's founding president, noted that "this was the first time that all the elements required to achieve a solution to the problem of doping in sport had come together, [including] the IOC, IFs, NOCs, athletes as well as intergovernmental organizations and national governments."[8]

Such a multilateral approach, in Pound's view, was the only path to a successful strategy; together, they could prove pessimists such as Samaranch wrong. "The fight against doping can not be won by the sports world alone," Pound later said. "There are many issues, such as the harmonization of legal penalties against doping, the trafficking of drugs and so forth that can only be resolved by the cooperative intervention of the governments of the world. That is why the World Anti-Doping Agency was created." Paraphrasing Winston Churchill's famous turn of words, Pound declared that in the struggle against pharmacological cheating one must "never give in, never give in, never[,] never, never. Never give in except to convictions of honour and good sense."[9]

Although de Merode possessed greater experience in anti-doping policy, he received little consideration for the position of WADA chair; Samaranch, according to Pound's later recollection, believed that de Merode no longer possessed the credibility requisite to effective leadership.[10] With both a law degree and certification as an accountant, Pound, on the other hand, was considered to be among the IOC's most effective administrators. Having played central roles in the formation of the IOC's successful marketing strategy and in the investigation of the Salt Lake City bribery scandal, he was a respected figure in both the Olympic and governmental communities.[11] A former elite swimmer, Pound believed deeply in the ideals espoused by the Olympic movement. Describing this philosophy, he wrote:

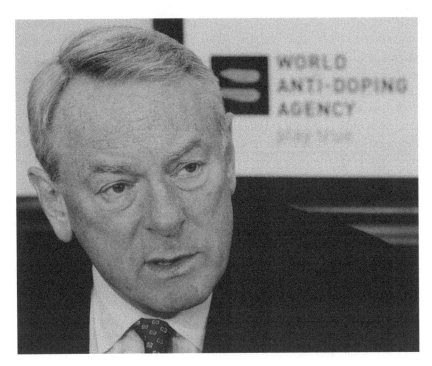

Montreal lawyer and chair of the World Anti-Doping Agency Dick Pound speaks during a news conference in Montreal, Canada, January 18, 2002 (ANDRE FORGET/AFP/Getty Images).

> I am convinced that the Olympic Games and the ethical prac-
> tice of sport are wonderful contributors to the organization
> of the youth of all countries. They assist in the development
> of social skills and abilities, and in the creation of a healthier
> society . . . that can make genuine contributions to peace in
> the world. I am, in that respect, a self-confessed and unrepen-
> tant idealist.[12]

If Pound had a weakness, it was an uncompromising personal style similar to that of Brundage. Unlike Brundage, however, Pound put his strong
leadership in the service of the anti-doping effort. Having been personally involved in the Ben Johnson crisis, he viewed drugs in athletics as a
"disease" that must be eliminated.[13] He was thus a near perfect match for
WADA's need of an aggressive, experienced leader.

Although WADA foundation board members agreed with the notion of a universal approach, they struggled to collectively identify a common set of short-term priorities. "The first thing that became clear to me when we started out," Pound later recalled, "was that when all is said and done[,] far more is said than done."[14] Some delegates accordingly focused on the "pharmacological arms race" between those who pursued new doping techniques and those seeking to catch them. Barry McCaffrey, a representative from the U.S. Office of National Drug Control Policy, argued, for example, that the agency should focus on developing a "gold standard" for the science of anti-doping. Optimistically asserting that the creation of WADA had effectively resolved the political fragmentation that had impaired previous efforts to control the proliferation of drugs in elite international athletics, he stated that the agency would be most effective through a rational "organization of science to deal with this complex problem." Having enormous confidence in the outcomes that could be produced in the type of private-public partnership that the agency exemplified, McCaffrey envisioned a quick resolution of the matter. "Doping," he declared, "was an easily resolvable issue in the coming decade if the science issue was focused upon."[15]

Those with more experience in the nuances of Olympic governance, however, realized that McCaffrey was blind to the deep-seated political, organizational, and legal problems that plagued the movement. "Once the agency was established," Pound later explained, "it became apparent quite early on that one of the greatest difficulties in the fight against doping in sport was the huge variations between the rules in different sports and different countries—and the level of their enforcement."[16] "The rules were all over the ballpark," he stated. "One sports organization had a life ban for the first positive test and another had a 2-week ban that you could serve between Christmas and New Year's."[17] Calling for a separation of elite sport from public judicial oversight, Paul Henderson, the International Sailing Federation's delegate to the foundation board meeting, similarly noted that "the biggest problem in the fight [against doping] was, upon finding a positive test, getting it upheld in the various levels of courts." He further stated that "there would have to be a major legal aspect to the body [WADA] to ensure that what was done was defended properly in the courts."[18] Henderson doubted that WADA would be ready to participate at the rapidly approaching 2000 Sydney Games, saying that "one hundred per cent of the responsibility for making sure that its athletes were clean lay with the country sending the athlete"; only at the conclusion of the competitions would WADA be in a position to assert itself.[19]

In the end, the board chose several points of emphasis for its first year.

Eschewing Henderson's warning against an overly demanding time line, the delegates decided to begin developing drug protocols in coordination with the various international federations for precompetition drug screens. Governments, they further decided, would be asked to increase their efforts to interdict the trafficking of illicit drugs in the time period preceding the opening of the Games. Most importantly, though, the board placed first priority on developing a universal set of anti-doping policies. A host of complex initiatives required coordination: developing the list of prohibited substances, accrediting testing laboratories, developing a doping results management system, and creating a new anti-doping code. Accordingly, the delegates declared that they would immediately "initiate the process of harmonizing anti-doping rules in sport and national legislation."[20] Two working groups were established as a result of the meeting; the first would begin review of a doping results management system for the competitions in Sydney, and the second would concentrate on drafting WADA's policies regarding conflicts of interests and public disclosure of the organization's activities.[21]

Pound, realizing that the development of such an ambitious program would take time, began the next meeting of the WADA foundation board by noting the considerable obstacles that would be faced in the nascent stages of such a large undertaking. Remarking that while efficiency was crucial, the delegates should make sure to "bear in mind that not all of WADA's objectives would be achieved at the current meeting and that it would take time for what were ambitious goals to be realized." Pound concluded that "the only way to eat an elephant was one bite at a time."[22] For issues that required immediate attention, the group, insisting that participation in Sydney was still realistic, concentrated on putting in place a precompetition protocol, to begin in April 2000. The absence of a detailed budget constrained future planning, although members expressed hope that the creation of an eleven-member executive board would streamline the agency's day-to-day operations. In order to strengthen the commitment of athletes to the anti-doping effort, an additional working group was created to consider the novel suggestion of a "doping passport" for Olympic competitors.[23]

WADA members hoped to provide some 10,000 drug screens before the opening of the events in Sydney, but the various international federations, which, after all, remained in control of the Olympic sports, still needed to be convinced of WADA's merits. Although optimistic regarding the plans for precompetition tests, WADA official Harri Syväsalmi feared, for example, that "we have very little time. We still have some job to do to persuade 15 federations to act on this issue."[24] As the opening of the Games neared, the obstacles presented by the Olympic regulatory structure became increasingly apparent. Indeed, by the June 2000 WADA executive committee meeting, the number of tests previously proposed had been reduced from 10,000 to 2,500.[25] The goal of autonomy for the agency was also proving elusive; the drug tests at the actual Olympic competitions would be conducted not by WADA, but through the other organizations in the international sport system.[26]

WADA executive board member Norman Moyer lamented that "the reason WADA had been created was precisely because the system in place had not delivered the level of credibility required."[27] Pound stressed that the process of consolidating authority in the new agency would not be quick or painless. He urged board members to maintain their course, bearing in mind that "WADA was a new organization dealing with IFs, which had their own autonomy." WADA should, Pound said, focus on what was realistically attainable in the few months before the competitions in Sydney commenced; afterward, members "could look at what had happened, and what could be done to improve things."[28]

2000 SYDNEY OLYMPIC GAMES

Despite the growing pains experienced by the agency, many policymakers believed that the Sydney Olympics would be the "cleanest" in the history of the movement. Rob Housman, the assistant director of strategic planning for the White House drug policy office, stated, for instance, that "there will be a new reality in Sydney. "Any athlete who is thinking about cheating," he elaborated, "has to think that if he does, he might get caught. Managing the tests and the results will be aboveboard and above reproach."[29] A new procedure for detecting instances of "blood doping" also gave hope to those who feared that novel performance-enhancing techniques might undermine the Games. Announcing a combined urine and blood screen for erythropoietin, Samaranch stated, "The scientists have decided that the tests may be implemented . . . I'm very optimistic because the panel [of experts recommending it] was unanimous."[30] IOC vice president Kevan Gosper was even more pleased: "I think," he declared, that "it will be a very good impact on the many athletes who do not cheat . . . For those who do cheat, I hope it scares the heck out of them."[31]

Concerned that the IOC might succeed in framing itself as the catalyst for the implementation of the tests, several WADA executive committee members worried that their future control over doping issues might be undermined. During an early August 2000 conference call, Canadian committee member Denis Coderre argued that "this kind of announcement on doping should be made by WADA itself," not by the IOC medical commission. "It was WADA," he said, "which should have the last word on whether tests such as these were performed or not. WADA's credibility was based on the word *world* in its title, which indicated that it [and not the IOC] enjoyed the trust of the people."[32] Advocating a less confrontational approach, Pound responded that the new screens should be welcomed with a strong endorsement by the agency. WADA, after all, did not yet have the political strength to openly contest the medical commission's authority. Pound again stressed to WADA members that the agency should bide its time, gradually establishing a broad base of support.[33]

To establish a presence at the Sydney Games, WADA instituted the Independent Observers Program, whose fifteen anti-doping experts would monitor the various doping control procedures at the competitions. Although prepared to state at the conclusion of the events that these were "the best Games ever," the body cited several problems in its postcompetition report. The ongoing diffusion that characterized the anti-doping framework of the movement was still troubling in that "issues were raised at times with respect to the I.O. [Independent Observer] role and its relation to the role of the IOC, its Medical Commission, and the Games Organising Committee." Describing the protectionist inclinations of a few members of the international sport community, the report continued that "it was not surprising that some considered the proposal one which could lead to interference with the work of the IOC's Medical Commission."[34] Athletes in Sydney were also bewildered by the increased number of anti-doping authorities there. Describing the precompetition screens sponsored by WADA, foundation board member Bob Ctvrtlik stated that while the competitors "were supportive of the programme in general . . . there had been some confusion between the different number of agencies that could test the athletes."[35]

Even though WADA was relegated to "observer" status at the Sydney Games, sports officials demonstrated their determination to implement an effective anti-doping program. The International Weightlifting Federation suspended the entire Romanian weightlifting team after several of its members failed drug screens prior to the Games.[36] During the actual competitions, the Bulgarian weightlifting team was told to leave after three of its lifters were disqualified for using prohibited diuretics.[37] As for WADA's first-year efforts, its out-of-competition testing program resulted in twenty-three positive indications of prohibited drug use.[38]

CONFLICT IN THE UNITED STATES

Fissures in the U.S. sports community contributed to the volatile environment that characterized the evolving Olympic anti-doping system. In the summer prior to the Sydney Games, Wade Exum, the director of the USOC's drug control program, resigned his position in part because he believed the committee was "deliberately encouraging" doping by U.S. competitors.[39] Combining this assertion with claims of racial discrimination on the part of the USOC, Exum filed a lawsuit in a U.S. federal district court alleging that approximately half of the instances in which athletes tested positive for performance-enhancing activities had not been addressed by the organization.[40] He further claimed that because the USOC implemented "absolutely no sanction" in many doping cases, such performance-enhancing substances as testosterone "continued to be routinely abused." As a result of this neglect, he continued, "the USOC actually encourages fringe performance enhancing and/or potential doping practices . . . on USOC premises." Exum further asserted that the "USOC's Drug Control program lacks a credible international and national reputation."[41] Responding to the accusations, USOC official Mike Moran asserted that any previous lapses in U.S. anti-doping efforts were, on the contrary, due to Exum's own incompetence. After all, Moran stated, Exum was the one in charge of the committee's anti-doping activities.[42]

A longstanding tension between international sports authorities and American officials also became apparent in Sydney as the former accused the latter of hypocrisy in their conduct concerning instances of doping by U.S athletes. Shortly before the opening of the Games, several members of the American swimming team blamed WADA for an unexplained drop in the number of drug screens at international events.[43] Matters were made worse when Barry McCaffrey, the U.S. national director of drug policy and a member of the WADA foundation board, refused to endorse a plan to underwrite WADA. "Since we already pay huge amounts of money to the IOC," he asked, "to what extent, if any, is additional funding required?" In response, Pound threatened to rescind the promise of governmental inclusion in the agency's decisions, commenting, "The deal is, if you want 50 percent of the seats on the board, you pay 50 percent of the pot."[44]

The accusations regarding the conduct of American officials arose from a perception that USA Track and Field (which governed the sport in America) was deliberately concealing positive drug screens by its athletes. When a report was published that shot-putter C. J. Hunter—husband of the famous American sprinter Marion Jones—had tested positive for the anabolic steroid nandrolone in July 2000, IOC officials criticized their American counterparts. Norwegian IOC delegate Gerhard Heiberg, having endured U.S. denigration of the IOC, accused American sports leaders of a double standard. "Yes, it's O.K. to criticize," he said, "[but] at the same time we feel your house is not in order. We feel you do not tell us the truth [about] what is happening in the United States." Heiberg continued, "You want us to be open instead of sweeping everything under the carpet. That has to go for the U.S. as well. We're a little irritated."[45] Dr. Arne Ljungqvist, serving as the chief medical officer of the International Amateur Athletic Federation, condemned USA Track and Field for failing to report in a timely fashion on a number of failed tests by athletes under its jurisdiction.[46] "We have no reason why," he said. "The Americans have taken the privilege on themselves to exonerate without informing us who [the athletes] are, and saying this is confidential."[47]

The disagreements between these rival national and international authorities quickly escalated to open discord among U.S. sports bodies. USA Track and Field leader Craig Masback, initially claiming that criticisms of his federation were "gratuitous shots from people who have no idea what the facts are," eventually asked WADA to assume command of his body's anti-doping efforts.[48] The U.S. Anti-Doping Agency (USADA) held the contract for these activities, and USADA chair Frank Shorter sarcastically commented, "Oh, so he wants USADA not to exist." He continued, "The ability to oversee testing is with the United States Olympic Committee . . . We have an agreement with the USOC to do their testing . . . You can only contract away rights that you have. USATF doesn't have the right to contract out the testing, because they've already given it away through the USOC to USADA."[49]

Perceiving an opportunity to consolidate WADA's authority over both national and international doping activities, Pound initially sided with Masback. "Ultimately," he stated, "that's probably the best way for all this to be played out—that all testing, for all national and international federations and national Olympic committees, be handled by an independent third party [WADA]."[50] When the WADA foundation board deliberated on the problem, however, Pound backpedaled, explaining that while he had a positive view of the idea, WADA was not yet in a position to assume the financial burden of the additional tests. Although the board endorsed a supervisory role for WADA in principle, it decided that—at least for the time being—the USA Track and Field protocols were best left in the hands of the USADA.[51] Two years later, though, Pound resumed his critique of American officials and even called for the expulsion of the U.S. track-and-field federation from the IAAF. "Kick them out," he said. "It's [anti-doping policy,] not rocket science. You can't have them flouting the rules."[52]

In the aftermath of the Sydney Games, the USOC was also quick to realize that it had to resolve the public controversy sparked by Exum's accusations that the committee had permitted drug usage among its athletes. Still perceiving the matter as a public relations issue rather than an ethical or organizational crisis, the USOC responded by instituting an expansive marketing campaign to reverse the damage. "Our image needs to be more clearly defined and brought to life in a compelling way for consumers," chief USOC marketing officer Matthew Mannelly declared. Elaborating on the effort, interim USOC chief executive officer Scott Blackmun added that "if we don't overcome the doping issue, the very basis that we distinguish ourselves from other sports properties disappears . . . All of a sudden, Olympic athletes are perceived as cheaters, which clearly, they are not."[53]

POST-SYDNEY DEVELOPMENTS

In the aftermath of the 2000 Summer Olympic Games, anti-doping policymakers focused on how best to address several organizational and scientific developments that were coming into play. Within WADA, a decision was made to increase the number of staff employees to keep pace with the goal of becoming the paramount international authority on the subject; for example, the need to maintain relations with public administrators led to the establishment of a new position for a government liaison officer.[54] Executive committee members, while pleased with the level of success that the agency had achieved in its first year of operation, remained worried by what they perceived to be an unwarranted focus on short-term matters. Looking over the program for the November 2000 committee meeting, for instance, Australian delegate Amanda Vanstone posited that she did not "see any discussion [scheduled] regarding where the Executive Committee wanted WADA to go, nor did the agenda indicate any strategy discussion. These were important issues." Even though the committee was entitled to "be almost euphoric with the achievements that WADA had made over the past 12 months, they now needed," she continued, "a strategy to take them up to [the 2002 Games in] Salt Lake City, in addition to a long-term strategy."[55]

WADA's still developing relationships with the international federations also required careful cultivation if the agency's out-of-competition testing program was to continue. Legal committee spokesperson David Howman identified a significant flaw in the new erythropoietin screens. "At present," he said, "very few IFs had the power within their constitution to conduct EPO blood testing, and for WADA to continue any out-of-competition testing with any emphasis on EPO testing, it would need to make sure that the IFs had their rules in place first." At a higher level, Howman continued, legal committee members "were also looking at making approaches to governments so that they could have in place protocols and ways of proceeding to allow out-of-competition testing to take place without complication." His committee thus "aimed to increase formal relationships with individual governments."[56]

At the same time, emerging developments in genetic science were creating a host of new issues for anti-doping policymakers. The anticipated completion of the mapping of the structure of human DNA through the Human Genome Project had the potential to eradicate a host of medical disorders that had plagued humankind since its beginnings, to facilitate criminal investigations, and to increase food sources for a growing world population.[57] Along with such benefits, however, came problems related to the possible application of genomics to elite athletics.[58] The IOC had long been aware of such prospects; describing the debates at the Centennial Olympic Congress held in 1994, IOC member Robert Parienté, for example, wrote that one question considered at the conference involved "how to prevent genetic manipulation . . . and thwart the maneuvers of those scientists who work for doping in greater numbers than those fighting against the scourge."[59] By now worried that new frontiers in performance enhancement were imminent, Olympic authorities planned a conference dedicated to a frank discussion of the matter. As put by IOC medical director Dr. Patrick Schamasch in May 2001, "For once we want to be ahead, not behind."[60] Lauding this cooperative approach, IAAF official Dr. Arne Ljungqvist stated, "For the first time, a substantial group of people involved in sports administration, sports science and genetic science will sit around the same table and discuss a common potential problem."[61] "The issue of gene therapy," he stated to the WADA executive committee, "was a very important one, and it was necessary to be prepared for when it arose."[62]

While some in the sports community perceived the ethical principles involved with genetic manipulation as easily resolvable, others were not so sure. U.S. Olympic champion Maurice Greene wondered, for instance, about the propriety of penalties in cases of prenatal or childhood applications of genetic enhancement; after all, he stated, "You [as an athlete] didn't have anything to do with it."[63] At a meeting held to discuss genomics in March 2002, Pound kept the focus on the main point that a firm stand should be taken regardless of philosophical arguments; under his conception, "sports are designed by people for people—people are not designed for a particular sport." In terms of substantive policies toward the subject, Pound asserted that new scientific techniques must be acquired. "The best way to deal with it," he declared, "is to prevent it and move quickly to the forefront of the technology."[64] At the same time, the increasing use of human growth hormone among elite athletes had not yet led to the development of an effective screen. Even when a test was implemented at the 2004 Athens Games, limitations regarding its "detection window" demonstrated the need for further scientific innovation.[65]

With the Olympics having instituted a new schedule during the 1990s in which the Summer and Winter Games alternated every two years, WADA stayed focused on bolstering its relative influence over doping issues in the short time remaining before the next competitions.[66] By the time the WADA executive board met in November 2000 in Oslo, seven of the international federations controlling winter sports had agreed to participate in the agency's out-of-competition testing program.[67] Still, much work needed to be done. Returning to the theme of coordinated action, board member Hein Verbruggen presented a damning critique of the earlier anti-doping framework, with its diffuse governance system:

> The problem was far too complex for the IFs to handle alone, and most IFs did not have the resources to perform tests or create education programmes. Also, the work done by the IFs was approximately 90% volunteer work. Previous research had been too scattered. The jurisdiction of the IFs was also far too limited for any decisive action where doping was concerned. [Verbruggen] therefore recommended that WADA have a role of coordination, harmonization, organization and supervision.[68]

Also realizing that WADA needed a permanent home if it was to become a credible organization, the agency initiated the process of identifying an acceptable location for its headquarters.[69] Because Lausanne, Switzerland, remained the IOC's host city, several executive committee members believed that it should be removed from consideration. Speaking at the November 2000 meeting of the IOC, Canadian representative Norman Moyer stated, "WADA had made an important point regarding the visible and real separation of WADA from the IOC, and it seemed . . . that the decision to locate the WADA headquarters in Lausanne was incompatible with the discussions that they had had around the table."[70] Supporting this conclusion, Coderre later stated that "if we really want to be efficient, neutral, independent and transparent, we cannot have in the same city the headquarters of the International Olympic Committee and the headquarters of the World Anti-Doping Agency."[71] Eventually, Montreal was chosen over five European-based competitors.[72]

Meanwhile, there were significant changes within the IOC leadership; Juan Antonio Samaranch retired in July 2001 with a decidedly mixed legacy. He had, on the one hand, steered the Olympics through the last years of the Cold War, during which the IOC's coffers were augmented by an unprecedented $12 billion in television revenues. Samaranch failed, however, to enact and enforce responsible, comprehensive doping reforms. Speaking to Samaranch's indifference toward the former GDR doping system, Australian IOC member Phil Coles remarked, for instance, that "that episode in sport was a black one."[73]

Upon Samaranch's retirement, the IOC had an opportunity to elect a leader who was more committed to anti-doping policy. The obvious choice was Dick Pound; as an IOC vice president, Pound had provided a strong voice for the creation of WADA, after which he served as its first chair. Pound, however, was "seen perhaps as too strong," said one anonymous IOC member. "He makes decisions without asking others."[74] A strong anti-American bias also worked against Pound, who, as a non-European, was perceived by some in the IOC as a mouthpiece for meddlesome North American policymakers.[75] While Pound did become a finalist, Belgian IOC member Jacques Rogge eventually won, in part because he advocated a less quarrelsome position toward such critical subjects as doping. "I think Jacques represents the right way to interpret the value of Olympism," said Italian IOC member Mario Pescante. "We need to stop a moment to reflect. Things have been running too fast in the past year."[76]

Fortunately, Rogge's victory was not altogether negative for the struggle against doping in the Olympic movement: first, the new president did have a more progressive outlook than Samaranch toward the need to resolve the doping problem; more importantly, Pound could remain in office at WADA. Once elected, Rogge, who was an orthopedic surgeon, certainly seemed enthusiastic about the medical reforms that were needed; in an editorial for the IOC's *Olympic Review,* he wrote, "Of the major problems that we must deal with, I must cite first of all the fight against doping and against corruption in sport."[77] Of course, such attestations of commitment had often been heard from previous IOC presidential administrations, including that of Samaranch. Rogge's sincerity was affirmed when he urged Pound to remain at WADA; "Dick has done an outstanding job as chairman of [the World Anti-Doping Agency]," he said, "and I think the continuation of his chairmanship is of a vital importance for the momentum that WADA has achieved now."[78]

Later remarking on such a surprising level of support by his former political opponent, Pound enthused, "One of the reasons I agreed to stay on in this position, I had a talk with Jacques and said this thing has to be driven by the IOC and WADA together, and if you are not 100 percent in favor it is not going to work . . . He said, 'I am 110 percent in favor' and he has been consistent and supportive." In comparing the new IOC president to Samaranch, Pound described Rogge's pragmatic approach as "the difference between the old school and the new school." For Samaranch, he continued, "a positive test was a failure in some way, a failure of the Olympics to be pure. The newer generation says, 'You don't understand, it is exactly the opposite. We have found someone cheating and taken that person out of the Games.' That is a successful program."[79] Progress in the fight against doping in Olympic competition required more than just individual leadership, however. National and international political dynamics remained crucial to the future of Olympic doping policy.

Thus far, national political units had acted primarily by pressuring private sports authorities to enact reform. Having succeeded in creating an entirely new regulatory framework for doping, it seemed possible that these units would now disengage from the problem—especially given their funding obligations to WADA. If the agency failed to finance its operations, the decades-long process of reform would end in disappointment.

Ten

DIFFICULTIES OF PARTNERSHIP

2002 SALT LAKE CITY GAMES

In January of 2002, news broke that a number of national governments had at last arranged to fulfill their funding obligations to WADA. With an additional $8.5 million from these sources, of which the U.S. and Canadian governments each contributed $800,000, the new agency expected that its yearly budget would grow to $25 million by 2006. The new erythropoietin screens cost between $1,000 and $1,200 each, and the additional funds allowed for a considerably more aggressive precompetition anti-doping program. As athletes grappled with the decision as to whether they should risk the tests by competing, Pound lauded the effort. "All of a sudden, a number of very important athletes around the world remembered they had left their iron on at home, and decided to stay there so there was no fire," he declared. "To me, that was a sign that it is a deterrent."[1] WADA confidently proclaimed that the Salt Lake City Olympics would be "the cleanest competition ever"—by now a familiar refrain.[2]

By the end of the month, WADA personnel had completed 2,600 of the anticipated 3,500 pre-Games drug screens (including over 200 erythropoietin tests), which collectively resulted in twenty-four positive indications of drug use.[3] The IOC remained in control of the tests conducted during the Winter Olympics, although WADA, serving as an independent oversight body, received an equal right of access to test results.[4] Focused on limiting costs, American officials in Salt Lake City perceived considerable fiscal inefficiency in the IOC's handling of drug testing. As president and CEO of the competition's organizing committee, Mitt Romney expressed particular dissatisfaction with de Merode's insistence on the construction of a doping laboratory at the competition site. Arguing at the time that an existing facility could more affordably conduct the tests, Romney later wrote that "we hated to have to spend the extra money for what some of us thought was the Prince's convenience."[5] Whatever the fairness of Romney's complaint, the friction resulting from the disagreement demonstrated that economic matters remained central to anti-doping decisions.

At the competitions, several skiers were suspended after an erythropoietin analogue called darbepoietin was found in their systems.[6] Weaknesses remained in the protocols, however, at least in the opinion of participating athletes. After Pavle Jovanovic, a member of the U.S. bobsled team, failed a doping screen and was suspended, American sled driver Todd Hays blamed anti-doping authorities for failing to provide enough information on nutritional supplements. "[The] USADA and the IOC is [sic] very knowledgeable about what's in these supplements," he argued. "The problem is, the IOC and USADA fail to educate us on this. Apparently, they test several hundred supplements and find 25 percent of them contain banned supplements. The problem is, they won't release the names of these companies."[7] When the case was heard on appeal, however, the Court of Arbitration for Sport found that Jovanovic was himself to blame for failing to consult anti-doping authorities on these issues.[8]

Although such incidents were less extensive than at many previous competitions, they continued to plague Olympic anti-doping authorities in Salt Lake City. Latvian bobsledder Sandis Prusis was permitted to participate in the Games even though he had tested positive for an anabolic steroid a year earlier; once again, the fragmented Olympic governance system was to blame. When WADA found traces of the prohibited agent nandrolone in his system during a November 2001 precompetition drug screen, Prusis received a three-month suspension from the International Bobsleigh and Skeleton Federation, which would expire six days before the first bobsled event in Utah. Alarmed that this lax approach would erode public confidence in the IOC, the IOC executive board declared Prusis ineligible to compete. After hearing the case on appeal, the Court of Arbitration for Sport overturned the IOC ruling, holding that international federations retained command of punitive measures for the athletes competing under their jurisdictions; in other words, the IOC could regulate federations but could not directly control federation decisions regarding individual athletes.[9] Angry at the result, Pound commented, "It's not fair, it's not right and it taints the performance of that athlete in the Games."[10]

Likewise, after Estonian cross-country skier Kristina Smigun's "A" specimen signaled the presence of norandrosteron in a December 2001 drug screen, a test of her "B" sample was automatically conducted at a different laboratory. When it failed to produce a similar positive result, rumors swirled that her screens had been illegally manipulated. Canadian national team coach David Wood sent an email to the International Ski Federation questioning the integrity of the protocols. "Is the testing process accurate or relevant?" he demanded. "Is the lab that conducted these tests incompetent, corrupt or both?"[11] Complicating the situation, the International Ski Federation rather than WADA held jurisdiction over the initial test, and athletes continued to express disappointment in the still fragmented doping control system. Writing to Pound, Canadian skier Beckie Scott asked, "Does it not seem just a little bit suspect . . . that the same organization we have been taking aim at for illegal behavior has now just conducted a test of their own that clears Kristina Smigun in time for the Olympics?"[12]

At the same time, WADA was affected by internal discord regarding its growing anti-doping initiatives. Beginning at the December 2001 executive committee meeting, disagreement arose as to the necessary components of the new erythropoietin screens. Committee member Hein Verbruggen, who was also a member of the IOC and president of the International Cycling Union, asserted that urine samples alone constituted an effective protocol; WADA scientists Arne Ljungqvist and Bengt Saltin argued, on the other hand, that blood specimens were also needed.[13] "It's beyond me," Verbruggen asserted, "why Bengt Saltin and Arne Ljungqvist didn't speak out earlier if UCI's urine test couldn't stand alone . . . To assert that the urine test is obsolete is a load of bullshit." Verbruggen, however, saved his most scathing remarks for Saltin: "He just sat on his fat arse for several months without saying a word until Nov[ember] 6 [2001] when WADA's medical commission, solely on the basis of Bengt Saltin's recommendation, submitted its proposal to the board for an Olympic EPO test consisting of a combination of urine samples and blood screens. I was speechless."[14]

Ljungqvist responded with an equal degree of contempt. "The argument against me and Bengt Saltin of having blocked urine-based EPO tests is idiotic," he said. "Verbruggen's theory of a conspiracy . . . against urine testing is absolutely ridiculous. He's very rude and has written threatening letters to both of us. I would only laugh at this if it were not a personal attack on my scientific integrity. It's irresponsible for an influential sports leader like Hein Verbruggen to do this, especially since his career is rising within the IOC."[15] After the competitions in Salt Lake City had concluded, the introduction of a new form of erythropoietin, which was difficult to distinguish from substances normally found in the human body, only made the situation worse. Disappointed at the corrosive effects of the argument, Pound remarked that the controversy was analogous to a situation in which "we sit in the car arguing while thieves are stealing the wheels."[16]

Another source of anxiety was that government funding for the new agency remained below the levels that had been originally promised. Addressing the tardiness of European payments at an international sport conference in Brussels, IOC director general François Carrard said, "There are some differences of opinion as to whether the European part of the budget should be financed by the [European Union] or by the individual [countries]. They failed to resolve this matter at the meeting and it will be discussed at a further meeting."[17]

Despite these problems, the anti-doping effort at the 2002 Olympic competitions was perceived as an important step toward the goal of creating a universal regulatory system. "I think Salt Lake City was a sign of how far we've come," said Pound. "Here the Russian cross-country skiers were using a new drug they thought no one could detect and they were laughing at us. Well, they're not laughing any more."[18] At the same time, however, the diffusion of anti-doping power remained a significant obstacle for policymakers. According to the WADA Independent Observers report for the Salt Lake City Games, for instance, the IOC's Anti-Doping Code conflicted with several passages of the Salt Lake City Doping Control Guide. The report accordingly recommended that "the protocols for blood collection and analysis must be harmonised and scientifically secure." Elaborating on the problems caused by the prevailing regime, the report noted that "competitors were still allowed to compete in skating events after a high blood count whereas, according to the [skiing] protocols, similar counts would have rendered them ineligible to compete in skiing events."[19]

THE PROCESS OF
POLITICAL UNIFICATION

In view of these remaining organizational problems, WADA advocated the creation of a new anti-doping code that, in contrast to the existing set of rules, would be universally applicable. IOC president Rogge, seeking to mend the longstanding rift between the medical committee and WADA, attended the opening of the permanent WADA headquarters in Montreal with promises of support. President Rogge, said WADA chief Dick Pound, "has been very supportive of WADA all along, far more unequivocal about his support than Samaranch ever would have been."[20] The WADA chair had also convinced a substantial number of sports leaders, including 200 national Olympic committees, 200 national governments, and 50 international federations, to endorse the agency's plan for a more robust anti-doping code.[21] Describing the anticipated effect of the agreement, Pound optimistically declared, "This is a tough code. If, by the [2004 Olympic] Games in Athens, you're not signed on, your country won't be there, or your sport won't be there. It's got teeth."[22]

The process of acquiring this degree of commitment from both private and public policymakers entailed several challenges. The outlines of the new code, first discussed at a December 2001 WADA executive committee meeting, were distributed at a series of international doping conferences over the next year, including the Harmonisation Congress in the Netherlands and, in Kuala Lumpur, the International Intergovernmental Consultative Group against Doping in Sport.[23] A complete version of the proposed code was presented to the WADA foundation board in June 2002 and was then subjected to an international review process. Over the next several months, two more drafts were written, circulated, and revised. After much work, the code was finally scheduled for presentation at the World Conference on Doping in Sport, which was to be held in March 2003 in Copenhagen.[24]

The subsequent adoption of the Copenhagen Declaration on Anti-Doping in Sport committed the world's leading athletic bodies to the regulatory structure embodied in the code. The code affirmed that "public authorities and sports organizations have complementary responsibilities to combat doping in sport" and that parties to the document "determined to take further and stronger cooperative action aimed at the reduction and eventual elimination of doping in sport."[25] In specifying the organizational elements of the new regulatory framework, the international agreement confirmed WADA's status as the supreme anti-doping authority; in a related measure, the signatories to the declaration pledged their support to the World Anti-Doping Code "as the foundation in the world wide fight against doping in sport."[26]

The adoption of the new WADA code was a promising development, but Pound, as he later wrote, understood that much work still needed to be done in terms of the implementation of the agreement. "It was little short of a miracle that the process had brought us this far this quickly," he remarked. "But WADA's adoption of the code was only the beginning. The code meant nothing until the sports movement and governments acted to incorporate it into their own rules."[27] To his credit, IOC president Rogge promised that adoption of the code was not to be considered optional. "There should be no place in the Olympic Games for international federations or national Olympic committees who refuse to implement the code," he said at the start of the Copenhagen conference. "Likewise," he continued, "no organization of the Olympic Games should be awarded to a country whose government has neglected or refused to implement the code."[28] The Copenhagen Declaration therefore called for the creation of an additional international convention that would bind national governments to its points; this document, under the declaration's time line, was to be adopted by the 2006 Winter Olympics.[29] Although the "binding" convention remained for future discussion, the Copenhagen conference took the single most important step in the history of Olympic doping policy: the creation of a universal regulatory system.

The IOC replaced its own medical code with the World Anti-Doping Code in July 2003, and pressure was subsequently placed on the various international federations to do the same by the opening of the 2004 Athens Olympic Games.[30] The International Cycling Union threatened to prohibit WADA's involvement at its 2003 world championships, using as its pretense an allegedly "leaked" document during that year's Tour de France. Pound promptly gave the ICU a deadline by which to adopt the WADA code. "There's a provision in the Olympic charter," he stated, "which by and large is hot off the press that says the world anti-doping code is obligatory for the whole Olympic movement." The International Cycling Union officials would, Pound declared, "have to adopt the code in the next 10 months."[31]

All that remained for the political unification of Olympic doping policy was an international convention that would formally bind national governments to the World Anti-Doping Code. The seeming indifference of the U.S. government to its financial role in the agency was particularly irksome to WADA officials. Pointing out that the United States—along with Italy and the Ukraine—had still not fulfilled its funding obligations, Pound asserted that the American team might face sanctions at the 2004 Summer Olympics; failure to fulfill its obligations might even cost New York the chance of hosting the 2012 Games. Of the George W. Bush administration, Pound said, "There's just a complete vacuum and void there as far as we're concerned."[32]

WADA pressed on, and the idea of the international convention was presented to the United Nations Educational, Scientific and Cultural Organization (UNESCO), where it was unanimously approved by all 191 member countries.[33] Proud that his government had been a leader in pushing for the international agreement, Stephen Owen, the Canadian minister of state with authority over athletics, declared, "The adoption of the convention will ensure that governments worldwide continue to work together to create an environment that enables athletes to compete on a fair and equal playing field."[34] The UNESCO International Convention against Doping in Sport, as the agreement was formally termed, would not come into effect, however, until at least thirty governments ratified it.[35] On November 25, 2005, Sweden became the first country to ratify the document; Pound hoped that twenty-nine more would do the same by the opening of the 2006 Winter Olympics in Torino, Italy.[36]

By February 2006, though, only seven national governments had ratified the convention. IOC president Rogge said, "We express the hope that the governments who have promised to adopt the code by the first day of the Olympic Games will accelerate their efforts."[37] Unfortunately, the goal was not met, and anti-doping authorities were consequently forced to deal with the issue in the absence of an enforceable treaty. The convention finally came into effect in February 2007.[38] Pound declared:

> [If] I was to say to you [when WADA was created in 1999
> that] within 5 years we're going to have an international code
> that will apply to all countries, all sports, in place, adopted
> by 202 national Olympic committees, 75 international sports
> federations, the IOC, and we'd have an international conven-
> tion under the umbrella of UNESCO unanimously approved,
> you'd look at me and say, "You're out of your mind."[39]

A NEW GOVERNMENTAL
INTEREST IN DOPING

Although at times it seemed that governments were not especially interested in doping policy, many, in fact, demonstrated high levels of commitment in the new politics of doping. Indeed, the anti-doping efforts of several governments were too aggressive for Olympic officials, who worried that they might destabilize the autonomy of the movement. A fine line thus existed, in the analysis of Olympic officials, between constructive public involvement and destructive political intrusion. Italy, for example, maintained legislation criminalizing doping in athletics, and the IOC sent a letter to the Italian government asking that the law be suspended for the Torino Games.[40]

Mario Pescante, an IOC member and Italian undersecretary for sport, sought a moratorium on the law, but the country's legislature refused to comply with the IOC's request. Pescante said, "Members of Parliament consider this moratorium a sign of weakness . . . I was very isolated."[41] Italian authorities did concede that IOC and WADA officials could conduct the in-competition drug screens. In addition, they suspended the authority of police forces to carry out random searches of athletes' quarters.[42] To some degree, then, national sovereignty over investigative procedures gave way to the wishes of international, nongovernmental sports authorities.

The U.S. Congress, recognizing the broader public policy implications, had repeatedly called for additional reforms along the WADA model.[43] President Bush even addressed doping in his 2004 State of the Union Address.[44] Bush's inclusion of anti-doping signaled the increasing strength of state partnership in anti-doping enforcement.

With the successful consolidation of anti-doping authority in WADA and its anti-doping code, combined with a more active stance on the part of governments, the next few years saw a growing number of criminal inquiries related to doping. Superstar sprinter Marion Jones received a six-month prison sentence for lying to federal authorities in their investigation of the Bay Area Laboratory Cooperative. At the private level, international sports authorities imposed a two-year suspension on Jones and revoked the five medals she won at the 2000 Sydney Games. John Fahey, the newly elected WADA president, remarked on the collaborative nature of these measures: "It is an example of how the work of WADA is making it more likely than ever that those who cheat in sport will be caught."[45] It remained unclear, however, whether the rising position of China in the international balance of power might trigger a return to the type of state involvement that existed during the Cold War, where governments that did not actively promote doping sometimes turned a blind eye to it.

BEIJING AND THE FUTURE

Historians addressing contemporary developments face a number of interpretive challenges. Despite the astounding amount of public information now available online, archival records pertaining to recent events in the Olympic movement remain largely unavailable. This appears to be especially true for documentary collections located in countries governed by authoritarian political regimes. In light of these evidentiary issues, a detailed analysis of the 2008 Summer Games in Beijing appears at this point unfeasible. Nevertheless, the available historical evidence points to several interesting developments in the international politics of doping.

Virtually every decision made by Chinese authorities regarding the 2008

Games reflected a broader set of internal and external priorities. In domestic affairs, the ruling Chinese Communist Party saw the competitions as a tool for strengthening national unity. Believing that internal division left China weak throughout most of the twentieth century, the Party leadership saw this outcome as being in the interests of the Chinese people. The fact that the domestic position of the Party would benefit in the process added force to their evaluation. At the international level, national leaders envisioned the Beijing Games as a statement of China's emergence at the center of world affairs.

In the context of these dynamics, many in the West feared a setback for anti-doping policy at the 2008 Beijing Games. Given the nature of the Chinese political regime, Western observers worried that the Chinese government might sponsor a doping program on the order of the Soviet and East German sport systems. Some remembered the almost comically inadequate procedures that were employed at the 1980 Games in Moscow. Some recalled that former Eastern-bloc coaches and scientists had found employment in China after the Cold War.[46] Western sports administrators also spoke of a new superpower conflict in Olympic competition. "In sporting terms, actually, we're all at war against China," said British Olympic official Simon Clegg.[47] Moreover, a series of Chinese drug scandals during the 1990s appeared to substantiate the existence of a state-sponsored doping program.

Although history may show otherwise, the available information suggests that these worries were overly pessimistic. To the contrary, Chinese officials greatly strengthened domestic anti-doping policies in the decade prior to the competitions. Broader international considerations lay behind these reforms, of course.[48] During the Cold War, policymakers calculated power in rather narrow military and economic terms. Having witnessed the disintegration of the Soviet empire, authorities in Beijing developed an alternative definition. On behalf of a "peaceful rise," they endeavored to demonstrate to the global community China's responsibility and commitment to nonviolence.

This model applied to the nation's behavior in international sport. Senior Chinese sports official Wang Wei declared in reference to this principle, "Winning the host rights to the 2008 Summer Games mean[t] winning the respect, trust, and favor of the international community."[49] A number of Western leaders held a similar vision. Former British prime minister Tony Blair argued in the *Wall Street Journal*, for instance, that the competitions provided a means to further bind the People's Republic to the international community. "These Games have given people a glimpse of modern China in a way that no amount of political speeches could do," he declared. "We can help China embrace the future."[50]

Reflecting similar beliefs, Chinese sports official He Zhenliang declared:

> The aim of China to participate in international competitions is to strengthen the friendship and mutual understanding . . . But, China does not need to establish her international position through several medals, she firmly refuses any medal tarnished by cheating . . . Chinese sports authorities will spare no effort to fight to the end against doping.[51]

The anti-doping structures employed in Beijing reflected these principles.

Prior to the competitions, IOC vice president Thomas Bach declared that in terms of testing for performance-enhancing substances, "The Beijing Games will be by far the most rigorously controlled ever and the most stringently controlled multi-sport event ever."[52] Scientific and ethical questions on doping remained, of course. Nevertheless, the apparently sincere response by Chinese leaders indicated that the political challenges involved in meeting the challenge of the doping problem continued to diminish. For the time being at least, international and national political currents seemed harmonious in their opposition to performance-enhancement in sport. The permanence of this unity remains a different question, of course.

CONCLUSION

Since doping first became an issue of public concern in the 1960s, Olympic policymakers, regardless of the individual organization to which they belonged, have for the most part confronted the problem on an ad-hoc basis with little long-term planning. For many years, substantive reforms were rarely undertaken outside times of crisis. This was in part due to the diffuse governance system under which the Olympic movement operates; until the establishment of WADA in 1999, regulatory power over doping was divided among several levels of international and national federations, national Olympic committees, and organizing bodies for individual competitions. And, up until the end of the Cold War, international political forces weighing against reform helped perpetuate the institutional fragmentation. Failures among public and private policymakers to recognize the saliency of doping and to fulfill their responsibilities for its effective regulation ensured that this structure would remain intact for multiple decades.

To be fair, there have been successes in the struggle to curtail performance-enhancing drugs in the Olympics, and not every individual in the Olympic community should be held personally culpable for the movement's failures. Few would argue, for example, that Dick Pound was willing to overlook controversial subjects for individual or organizational gain. Nevertheless, Olympic leaders with Pound's integrity remained far too few for much too long. IOC president Avery Brundage was too enmeshed in notions of amateurism to spend much time on "insignificant" matters like doping; his successor, Lord Killanin, bumbled his way through eight years of leadership, accomplishing little; perhaps worst of all, Juan Antonio Samaranch chose for the most part to ignore the issue, focusing his attention on the economic growth of the Olympic movement. Even during the past decade, those willing to take a stand against the status quo have often been punished. Dick Pound's support of an aggressive anti-doping mechanism very likely led to his third-place finish in the 2001 IOC presidential election. Indeed, a combination of organizational decentralization, venality, and individual indifference have seriously diminished the likelihood of an effective and sustained anti-doping policy.

Even when progress was made, plans for reform were usually prepared only after the occurrence of some "focusing event" that frightened policymakers into action. This shortcoming was perhaps best articulated at a November 2000 meeting of the WADA foundation board by member Paul Henderson, who observed, "No good lesson was ever learnt except through the eyes of disaster."[1] People knew that athletes were using performance-enhancing drugs prior to Knud Jensen's death in 1960, for example, but serious dialogue did not begin until after that event. And, while regulations against doping were gradually instituted over the next decade, the powers to enforce them remained dispersed among the various components of the movement's governance system.

Despite periodic efforts at altering the status quo, this decentralized anti-doping framework was maintained until the last stages of the Cold War. In response to the changed international environment, public authorities reacted swiftly after Canadian sprinter Ben Johnson tested positive for an anabolic steroid at the 1988 Summer Olympics in Seoul, South Korea. Facing the specter of government intervention, Olympic policymakers were spurred to action. Even so, it took policymakers over a decade to implement a more integrated regime through the creation of the World Anti-Doping Agency in November 1999.

To their credit, anti-doping authorities, freed from the previously fragmented regulatory system with the creation of WADA and the ratification of the World Anti-Doping Code, began to plan for the scientific advances that would collectively constitute the future of doping. During the first decade of the twenty-first century, for example, a succession of international conferences took place regarding the possible applications of genomics to athletic enhancement. Speaking to the anticipated benefits of this early start, WADA member Theodore Friedmann asserted, "There is a much greater level of awareness, and that's the starting point."[2] The World Anti-Doping Code even included a provision that "the use of genetic transfer technology to dramatically enhance sport performance should be prohibited as contrary to the spirit of sport even if it is not harmful."[3]

The tragedy is that however admirable, these developments occurred too late to definitively "win" the war against doping in the Olympics. The fact is that we live in a performance-enhanced society. Examples of this abound: the stimulant Dexedrine was used by military pilots in the Gulf

War of 1990, college students regularly take amphetamine-based drugs in pursuit of higher grade-point averages, and an increasing number of non-elderly individuals are prescribed testosterone and human growth hormone to counteract the effects of aging.[4] In the Olympics, this "medicalized" environment has led to accepted forms and levels of "soft doping." Under current WADA guidelines, for example, a competitor's testosterone to epi-testosterone ratio must exceed 4.0 before a urine sample is submitted to iso-topic ratio mass spectrometry. Given that this ratio far exceeds that which is ordinarily found in the human body, athletes are effectively allowed to "cheat" within arbitrarily constructed limits.[5] The resulting uncertainty as to the legitimacy of the drug screens used by sports authorities worries a growing number of exercise scientists.[6] The genetic revolution will only make matters worse; alluding to novelist Aldous Huxley's gloomy vision of the human future, Pound thus stated, "The drug problem is the devil we know . . . and here we are at the beginning of a brave new world."[7]

The dilemmas presented by these prospects were perhaps best articu-lated in March 2002 by Joseph Glorioso, director of the Pittsburgh Hu-man Gene Therapy Center, in a question that cut to the heart of the fu-ture of doping. "How do we distinguish enhancement from treatment?" he wondered.[8] Elucidating the answer will be the central challenge for future Olympic policymakers.

NOTES

INTRODUCTION

1. The few diplomatic historians who have written on the subject have done so largely for public rather than academic audiences. Even when sophisticated interpretations have been produced, they have been supported almost entirely by non-archival sources of information. One example of this type of literature is Walter LaFeber's *Michael Jordan and the New Global Capitalism*, expanded ed. (New York: Norton, 2002). See also Thomas W. Zeiler, *Ambassadors in Pinstripes: The Spalding World Baseball Tour and the Birth of the American Empire* (Lanham, MD: Rowman and Littlefield, 2006). Barbara Keys's *Globalizing Sport: National Rivalry and International Community in the 1930s* (Cambridge, MA: Harvard University Press, 2006) serves as the first truly significant study on sport published by a diplomatic historian.

2. Those political scientists who have published on the topic have done so outside the boundaries of international relations theory. See, for one example, Derick L. Hulme, *The Political Olympics: Moscow, Afghanistan, and the 1980 U.S. Boycott* (New York: Praeger, 1990). Although their theoretical efforts remain embryonic, a small number of political scientists have very recently begun to reverse this trend. See, for example, Victor D. Cha, *Beyond the Final Score: The Politics of Sport in Asia* (New York: Columbia University Press, 2009).

3. See, on this point, notes 8 and 15 of Steven W. Pope, "Rethinking Sport, Empire, and American Exceptionalism," *Sport History Review* 38 (2007): 110, 111. Among the few sport historians who have produced significant interpretations of sport and international relations, the most noteworthy remains Mark Dyreson, who wrote a seminal study on the use of international sport as a nation-building mechanism in the United States. See his *Making the American Team: Sport, Culture, and the Olympic Experience* (Champagne: University of Illinois Press, 1998). See also Dyreson, "Globalizing the Nation-Making Process: Modern Sport in World History," *International Journal of the History of Sport* 20 (March 2003): 91–106. Other important exceptions include Allen Guttmann's early study of sport and imperialism: *Games and Empires: Modern Sports and Cultural Imperialism* (New York: Columbia University Press, 1996); Alan M. Klein's *Sugarball: The American Game, the Dominican Dream* (New Haven, CT: Yale University Press, 1991); Klein, *Growing the Game: The Globalization of Major League Baseball,* reprint ed. (New Haven, CT: Yale University Press, 2008); and Gerald Gems,

The Athletic Crusade: Sport and American Cultural Imperialism (Lincoln: University of Nebraska Press, 2006).

4. Cha, *Beyond the Final Score*, 30.

5. The significant early works include Terry Todd, "Anabolic Steroids: The Gremlins of Sport," *Journal of Sport History* 14, no. 1 (Spring 1987): 87–107; Todd, "A History of the Use of Anabolic Steroids in Sport," in *Sport and Exercise Science: Essays in the History of Sports Medicine*, edited by Jack W. Berryman and Roberta J. Park (Urbana: University of Illinois Press, 1992); Charles E. Yesalis, ed., *Anabolic Steroids in Sport and Exercise*, 2nd ed. (Champaign, IL: Human Kinetics, 2000); Charles Yesalis and Virginia S. Cowart, *The Steroids Game* (Champaign, IL: Human Kinetics, 1998); Wayne Wilson and Edward Derse, eds., *Doping in Elite Sport: The Politics of Drugs in the Olympic Movement* (Champaign, IL: Human Kinetics, 2001), especially the chapter by Todd and Todd, "Significant Events in the History of Drug Testing and the Olympic Movement: 1960–1999," 65–128. John M. Hoberman has written the leading works on the subject. See his *Mortal Engines: The Science of Performance and the Dehumanization of Sport* (New York: Free Press, 1992) and *Testosterone Dreams: Rejuvenation, Aphrodisia, Doping* (Berkeley: University of California Press, 2005). A perceptive overview of Hoberman's influence on how scholars currently understand performance enhancement in sport is provided by Paul Dimeo in "A Critical Assessment of John Hoberman's Histories of Drugs in Sport," *Sport in History* 27, no. 2 (June 2007): 318–342.

6. Paul Dimeo's *A History of Drug Use in Sport, 1876–1976: Beyond Good and Evil* (New York: Routledge, 2007), however, began to redress this situation by utilizing primary sources of evidence.

7. See Andy Miah, *Genetically Modified Athletes: Biomedical Ethics, Gene Doping and Sport* (New York: Routledge, 2005); Dimeo, *A History of Drug Use in Sport;* and Hoberman, *Mortal Engines* and *Testosterone Dreams,* though the latter two volumes cover politics as well.

8. For the idea of an autonomous international sport community, see Keys, *Globalizing Sport.*

9. The complex relationship between nation-states and the private international anti-doping regime is captured in Barrie Houlihan, "Mechanisms of International Influence on Domestic Elite Sport Policy," *International Journal of Sport Policy* 1 (March 2009): 59–61.

10. For the belief that sport could inspire a sense of patriotism, see Mark Dyreson, *Crafting Patriotism for Global Dominance: America at the Olympics* (New York: Routledge, 2009).

11. A water polo match between the Soviet and Hungarian teams in the 1956 Summer Olympic Games, during the Hungarian uprising against Soviet control, served as an early indicator of the place of sport in Eastern-bloc resistance against the Soviet Union. See Robert E. Rinehart, "Cold War Expatriot Sport: Symbolic Resistance and International Response in Hungarian Water Polo at the Melbourne Olympics, 1956," in *East Plays West: Sport and the Cold War*, ed. Stephen Wagg and David L. Andrews (New York: Routledge, 2007), 45–63. The employment of sport for nationalist purposes varied across the Soviet satellite system. As Thierry Terret notes, "The relations between Sofia and Moscow had nothing in common with the much more problematic ones that pertained between Budapest and the Russian capital after the events of 1956."

Terret, "Sport in Eastern Europe during the Cold War," *International Journal of the History of Sport* 26, no. 4 (March 2009): 466.

12. On this point, consult Dionne Koller, "From Medals to Morality: Sportive Nationalism and the Problem of Doping in Sports," *Marquette Sports Law Review* 19, no. 1 (Fall 2008): 91–124; Koller, "How the United States Government Sacrifices Athletes' Constitutional Rights in Pursuit of National Prestige," *Brigham Young University Law Review* (Fall 2008): 1465–1544. On the connection between doping in international sport and the Cold War, see Thomas M. Hunt, "Sport, Drugs, and the Cold War: The Conundrum of Olympic Doping Policy, 1970–1979," *Olympika: The International Journal of Olympic Studies* 16 (2007): 19–42.

13. The medical priorities of the Olympic community during the 1960s are elaborated in Allan J. Ryan, "A Medical History of the Olympic Games," *Journal of the American Medical Association* 205 (September 9, 1968): 715–720.

14. Quote from "Letter from the Publisher," *Sports Illustrated,* June 23, 1969, 4. A more accessible source for this quote is Todd and Todd, "Significant Events in the History of Drug Testing and the Olympic Movement," 70. See also Bil Gilbert, "Drugs in Sport: Problems in a Turned On World," *Sports Illustrated,* June 23, 1969, 64–72; Gilbert, "Drugs in Sport: Something Extra on the Ball," *Sports Illustrated,* June 30, 1969, 31–32, 37–40; and Gilbert, "Drugs in Sport: High Time to Make Some Rules," *Sports Illustrated,* July 7, 1969.

15. See Koller, "From Medals to Morality." The evolution of state involvement in doping during the late 1980s is also discussed in Maxwell J. Mehlman, Elizabeth Banger, and Matthew M. Wright, "Doping in Sports and the Use of State Power," *St. Louis University Law Journal* 15 (2005/2006): 15–73.

16. An excellent description of focusing events is provided in John W. Kingdon, *Agendas, Alternatives, and Public Policies,* 2nd ed. (New York: Longman, 2003), 94–100.

17. At least one study argues that governmental intervention in doping questions served as the primary agent in changing the existing regulatory framework. See Dag Vidar Hanstad, Andy Smith, and Ivan Waddington, "The Establishment of the World Anti-Doping Agency: A Study of the Management of Organizational Change and Unplanned Outcomes," *International Review for the Sociology of Sport* 43, no. 3 (September 2008): 227–249.

18. For the longstanding diffusion of anti-doping powers and the drive toward a centralized approach, see Barrie Houlihan, "Policy Harmonization: The Example of Global Antidoping Policy," *Journal of Sport Management* 13 (July 1999): 197–215.

CHAPTER 1

1. "Inquiry to Last Several Weeks: Use of Roniacol Is Blamed for Death of Knud Jensen in Olympic Bike Race," *New York Times,* August 30, 1960.

2. "L.A. Cyclist Says Other Nations Used Stimulants," *Los Angeles Times,* August 30, 1960.

3. "Inquiry to Last Several Weeks."

4. "Trainer Says He Issued Cyclist Drug," *Chicago Daily Tribune,* August 29, 1960.

5. Australian Broadcasting Corporation webpage dated March 17, 2003, http://www.abc.net.au/cycling/items/s809238.htm. A contemporaneous newspaper report disputes the findings of the autopsy: "Find No Drug in Olympics Cycling Death," *Chicago Daily Tribune,* March 26, 1961. The lack of substantive corroboration that Jensen ingested amphetamines is detailed in Verner Møller, "Knud Enemark Jensen's Death during the 1960 Rome Olympics: A Search for Truth?" *Sport in History* 25, no. 3 (December 2005): 452–471.

6. "Sportive nationalism" is a concept borrowed from John Hoberman. See especially *Testosterone Dreams,* 249–260.

7. Brundage quoted in Paul Gardner, "Dope," magazine clipping, Avery Brundage Collection (microfilm edition; originals located at the University of Illinois at Urbana-Champaign Archives), Box 99, Folder "SP Medical Commission, IOC, 1966–1969," p. 37.

8. Gaston Mullegg and Henry Montandon, "The Danish Oarsm[e]n Who Took Part in the European Championships at Milan in 1950: Were They Drugged?" *Bulletin du Comité International Olympique,* July 1951, 26. For this and other references to doping in the IOC *Bulletin* around this time, see also Alison M. Wrynn, "The Human Factor: Science, Medicine and the International Olympic Committee, 1900–70," *Sport in Society* 7, no. 2 (Summer 2004): 217. A brief overview of early IOC doping policies is additionally provided in Raymond Gafner, ed., *1894–1994, The International Olympic Committee: One Hundred Years—The Idea—The Presidents—The Achievements,* vol. 2 (Lausanne: International Olympic Committee, 1994), 165–167.

9. "After the Congress of the Association Internationale de Boxe Amateur," *Bulletin du Comité International Olympique,* September 1951, 16.

10. See Houlihan, *Dying to Win: Doping in Sport and the Development of Anti-Doping Policy,* 2nd ed. (Strasbourg, France: Council of Europe Publishing, 2002), 34.

11. Hoffman quoted in Elliott Almond, Julie Cart, and Randy Harvey, "Testing Has Not Stopped Use of Steroids in Athletics: Soviets Led the Way, but West Has Caught Up," *Los Angeles Times,* January 29, 1984.

12. Ziegler quoted in John D. Fair, "Isometrics or Steroids? Exploring New Frontiers of Strength in the Early 1960s," *Journal of Sport History* 20, no. 1 (Spring 1993): 4.

13. For these experiments, see Fair, "Isometrics or Steroids?" 5–6.

14. See Todd, "A History of the Use of Anabolic Steroids in Sport," 325–326. For a discussion of research regarding the removal of testosterone's androgenic properties while keeping its anabolic benefits, see Charles D. Kochakian and Charles E. Yesalis, "Anabolic-Androgenic Steroids: A Historical Perspective and Definition," in *Anabolic Steroids in Sport and Exercise,* ed. Charles E. Yesalis, 2nd ed. (Champaign, IL: Human Kinetics, 2000), 26–30.

15. Richard W. Pound, *Inside the Olympics: A Behind-the-Scenes Look at the Politics, the Scandals, and the Glory of the Games* (Etobicoke, ON: J. Wiley & Sons Canada, 2004), 54–55. Pound was a member of the Canadian Olympic swimming team when he heard these rumors. He later became vice president of the IOC and then president of the World Anti-Doping Agency (WADA). While head of WADA, Pound elaborated his moral conception of the doping problem in *Inside Dope: How Drugs Are the Biggest Threat to Sports, Why You Should Care, and What Can Be Done about Them* (Mississauga, ON: John Wiley & Sons Canada, 2006).

16. British Olympic official Sir Adolphe Abrahams asserted, for instance, that Bannister's run "owes nothing to amphetamine (or any other drug)." In the United States, the National Collegiate Track Coaches Association released a statement criticizing "the unwarranted and unsubstantiated statements . . . [attributing] the development in track and field athletics to the indiscriminate use of harmful drugs, specifically compounds of Benzedrine. We who are connected with track know that this statement is contrary to fact." For the debate over doping in the context of Bannister's run, consult John M. Hoberman, "Amphetamine and the Four-Minute Mile," *Sport in History* 26, no. 2 (August 2006): 289–304. Quotes provided in this footnote are from pages 290–291 of Hoberman's article.

17. H. H. Pius XII, "Let Us Condemn the Practice of Doping," *Bulletin du Comité International Olympique,* February 1956, 65.

18. Avery Brundage to Henry Beecher, January 9, 1960, Avery Brundage Collection, Box 99, Folder "SP Medical IOC Amphetamines Used in Athletics, 1937–1969." The three articles that Beecher sent Brundage were as follows: Allan J. Ryan, "Use of Amphetamines in Athletics," *Journal of the American Medical Association* 170 (May 30, 1959): 562; Peter V. Karpovich, "Effect of Amphetamine Sulfate on Athletic Performance," *Journal of the American Medical Association* 170 (May 30, 1959): 558–561; Gene M. Smith and Henry K. Beecher, "Amphetamine Sulfate and Athletic Performance," *Journal of the American Medical Association* 170 (May 30, 1959): 543–557. Avery Brundage Collection, Box 99, Folder "SP Medical IOC Amphetamines Used in Athletics, 1937–1969."

19. Minutes of the General Session of the International Olympic Committee, February 1960, San Francisco, International Olympic Committee Library, Lausanne (hereafter IOCL), p. 9. For the point concerning Brundage's focus on amateurism rather than doping, see Allen Guttmann, *The Games Must Go On: Avery Brundage and the Olympic Movement* (New York: Columbia University Press, 1984), 123.

20. Todd and Todd, "Significant Events in the History of Drug Testing and the Olympic Movement: 1960–1999," 66. The Todds mention Eklund's proposed investigation, citing Wolf Lyberg (a former IOC member), *The IOC Sessions: 1956–1988, Volume 2—A Study Made by Wolf Lyberg, Former Secretary General of the NOC of Sweden,* n.p., n.d., p. 46. The official minutes of the meeting, however, do not mention this claim. The IOC's proposal can be found in Minutes of the IOC General Session, February 1960, San Francisco, IOCL, p. 9.

21. Danish scholar Verner Møller notes that prior to the 1960s, "a rather liberal attitude toward the use of performance-enhancing substances had prevailed." See his *The Doping Evil,* translated by John M. Hoberman (Copenhagen: Books on Demand GmbH, 2008), 33. This text was originally published in 1999 as "Dopingdjævlen— analyse af en hed debat." Translated and reprinted by permission of the publishers, Gyldendal, Denmark. The English version is available online at http://www.scribd .com/doc/14022659/The-Doping-Devil. Daniel M. Rosen, writing for a popular audience, asserts that scandals in the 1950s changed society's conceptions of doping. See his *Dope: A History of Performance Enhancement in Sports from the Nineteenth Century to Today* (Westport, CT: Praeger, 2008), 1–21. These pages provide an accessible overview of the early history of performance-enhancing substances. See also Dimeo, *A History of Drug Use in Sport, 1876–1976.*

22. Lucas quoted in Dyreson, *Making the American Team,* 89. For historical context on Hicks, see John M. Hoberman, "History and Prevalence of Doping in the Marathon," *Sports Medicine* 37, no. 4/5 (2007): 366–388.

23. Lucas quoted in Allen Guttmann, *The Olympics: A History of the Modern Games,* 2nd ed. (Urbana: University of Illinois Press, 2002), 27. The best recent analysis of Hicks and the 1904 Olympic marathon is provided by Paul Dimeo in his *A History of Drug Use in Sport, 1876–1976,* 25–27. Those interested in the larger context of the 1904 Games should consult George R. Matthews, *America's First Olympics: The St. Louis Games of 1904* (Columbia: University of Missouri Press, 2005), though it sheds little light on the Hicks episode.

24. Lucas quoted in Dyreson, *Making the American Team,* 90.

25. Avery Brundage to Otto Mayer, November 10, 1960, referenced in Alison Wrynn, "The Human Factor: Science, Medicine and the International Olympic Committee, 1900–70," *Sport in Society* 7, no. 2 (Summer 2004): 218.

26. Minutes of the Meetings of the Executive Board of the International Olympic Committee, September 10, 1960, Rome, IOCL, p. 3.

27. Minutes of the IOC Executive Board, June 15, 1961, Athens, IOCL, p. 2.

28. Minutes of the IOC General Session, June 1961, Athens, IOCL, p. 3.

29. Avery Brundage to Otto Mayer, January 8, 1962, quoted in Wrynn, "The Human Factor," 218.

30. "Speech Given by Mr. Avery Brundage, President of the International Olympic Committee, June 23, 1964, at la Sorbonne in Paris," *Bulletin du Comité International Olympique,* August 1964, 48.

31. For Brundage's involvement in the American debate over a 1936 boycott, consult Carolyn Marvin, "Avery Brundage and American Participation in the 1936 Olympic Games," *Journal of American Studies* 16, no. 1 (April 1982): 81–105.

32. Porritt and Van Karnebeek quoted in Allen Guttmann, *The Games Must Go On,* 112.

33. Jeremiah Tax, "An In-Depth Look at Both the Seemly and Seamy Sides of Avery Brundage," *Sports Illustrated,* January 16, 1984.

34. The best biography of Brundage is Guttmann, *The Games Must Go On.* This work provides particularly excellent discussions of his philosophy regarding sport.

35. Original in French. Proces-Verbal de la réunion de la Commission Exécutive du C.I.O avec la Commission d'Amateurisme, March, 3, 1962, Lausanne, IOCL, p. 3. For more on the IOC's relationship with the FIMS, see Wrynn, "The Human Factor," 213.

36. Arthur Porritt, "Report on a Proposed Scientific Congress regarding Medical Sporting Questions," IOC General Session, January 1948, St. Moritz, Switzerland, quoted in Wrynn, "The Human Factor," 213.

37. Otto Mayer to Kyotaro Asuma and Arthur Porritt, March 12, 1962, Avery Brundage Collection, Box 99, Folder "SP Medical IOC Amphetamines Used in Athletics, 1937–1969."

38. Otto Mayer to the Members of the Commission of Doping, April 21, 1962, Avery Brundage Collection, Box 99, Folder "SP Medical IOC Amphetamines Used in Athletics, 1937–1969."

39. Mayer to Porritt, April 12, 1962, Avery Brundage Collection, Box 99, Folder "SP Medical IOC Amphetamines Used in Athletics, 1937–1969."

40. Mayer to Porritt, April 3, 1962, Avery Brundage Collection, Box 99, Folder "SP Medical IOC Amphetamines Used in Athletics, 1937–1969."

41. Minutes of the IOC General Session, June 1962, Moscow, IOCL, p. 4.

42. Mayer to Porritt, September 27, 1962, Avery Brundage Papers, Box 99, Folder "SP Medical IOC Amphetamines Used in Athletics, 1937–1969."

43. Porritt to Mayer, October, 23, 1962, Avery Brundage Collection, Box 99, Folder "SP Medical IOC Amphetamines Used in Athletics, 1937–1969." Referring again to his commitment to other concerns, Porritt later wrote to Brundage that "it is good of you to let me off my Chairmanship of the Doping Commission but I really have tried to find time to do this but, at the moment, am just stymied." Porritt to Brundage, November 5, 1962, Avery Brundage Collection, Box 99, Folder "SP Medical IOC Amphetamines Used in Athletics, 1937–1969." Given Porritt's stance in regard to scientific questions and Brundage's reluctance to deal with doping issues, one wonders whether the IOC president chose Porritt as chair of the new commission in order to slow policy development on the subject.

44. Avery Brundage to Porritt, November 1, 1962, Avery Brundage Collection, Box 99, Folder "SP Medical IOC Amphetamines Used in Athletics, 1937–1969."

45. J. Ferreira Santos and Mario de Carvalho Pini, "Doping," *Bulletin du Comité International Olympique,* February 1963, 56. The definition of doping as "illegal" in this article illustrates the conceptual difficulty that the IOC experienced in coming to grips with the subject. Although certain nations have in recent decades made the use of performance-enhancing substances in athletic competitions a crime, Olympic leaders have consistently fought against this type of governmental involvement. For the use of criminal penalties for doping offenses, see Christopher McKenzie, "The Use of Criminal Justice Mechanisms to Combat Doping in Sport," *Bond University Sports Law eJournal* (August 2007), http://epublications.bond.edu.au/slej/4/.

46. Brundage to Mayer, February 26, 1963, quoted in Wrynn, "The Human Factor," 218.

47. "The Anti-Doping Battle Is Making Good Progress," *Bulletin du Comité International Olympique,* May 1963, 43–44. See also Todd and Todd, "Significant Events in the History of Drug Testing and the Olympic Movement," 67.

48. "Doping, the International Olympic Committee and the Press," *Bulletin du Comité International Olympique,* November 1963, 60.

49. Minutes of the IOC General Session, January 1964, Innsbruck, IOCL, pp. 12–13.

50. Minutes of the IOC Executive Board, October 16, 1964, Tokyo, IOCL, p. 1.

51. U.S. Senate, Committee on the Judiciary, Subcommittee to Investigate Juvenile Delinquency of the Committee on the Judiciary, *Investigative Hearings on the Proper and Improper Use of Drugs by Athletes before the Subcommittee to Investigate Juvenile Delinquency of the Committee on the Judiciary Pursuant to S. Res. 56, Section 12.,* 93rd Congress, 1st sess., June 18, July 12, 13, 1973 (Washington, DC: U.S. Government Printing Office, 1973), 274.

52. See Wrynn, "The Human Factor," 219.

53. Minutes of the Meeting of the IOC Executive Board, October 16, 1964, Tokyo, IOCL, p. 1.

54. Minutes of the IOC General Session, October 1964, Tokyo, IOCL, p. 11.

55. See Alison M. Wrynn, "'A Debt Was Paid Off in Tears': Science, IOC Poli-

tics and the Debate about High Altitude in the 1968 Mexico City Olympics," *International Journal of the History of Sport* 23, no. 7 (November 2006): 1152–1172. See also Kevin B. Witherspoon, *Before the Eyes of the World: Mexico and the 1968 Olympic Games* (DeKalb: Northern Illinois University Press, 2008), 48–55. Ethicists, physicians, and policymakers continue to debate the connection between altitude training and doping, especially after "artificial" hypoxic environments began to be used. For a medical argument against defining their use as doping, see Benjamin D. Levine, "Should 'Artificial' High Altitude Environments Be Considered Doping?" *Scandinavian Journal of Medicine and Science in Sports* 16, no. 5 (October 2006): 297–301. For a recent review of how altitude training increases athletic performance, see Aurelie Gaudard, Emmanuelle Varlet-Marie, Francoise Bressolle, and Michel Audran, "Drugs for Increasing Oxygen Transport and Their Potential Use in Doping: A Review," *Sports Medicine* 33, no. 3 (2003): 191–193. For a philosophical argument against altitude training—or any other technique—as doping, see J. Salvulescu, B. Foddy, and M. Clayton, "Why We Should Allow Performance Enhancing Drugs in Sport," *British Journal of Sports Medicine* 38, no. 6 (December 2004): 666–670.

56. For recollections of the 1955 Pan-American Games in the Mexican Capital, see Witherspoon, *Before the Eyes of the World*, 50.

57. Minutes of the IOC General Session, October 1963, Lausanne, IOCL, p. 6.

58. Minutes of the IOC General Session, October 1964, Tokyo, IOCL, p. 11.

59. Wrynn, "'A Debt Was Paid Off in Tears,'" 1156. See also Witherspoon, *Before the Eyes of the World*, 50.

60. Wrynn, "'A Debt Was Paid Off in Tears,'" 1156.

61. Minutes of the IOC General Session, October 1963, Baden-Baden, IOCL, p. 6.

62. Minutes of the Meeting of the Board of Directors of the United States Olympic Committee, May 3–4, 1964, New York, United States Olympic Committee Library and Archives (hereafter USOCLA), pp. 55, 54.

63. Wilson and McPhee quoted in Minutes of the USOC Board of Directors, March 22–23, 1965, New York, USOCLA, p. 73.

64. Minutes of the USOC Board of Directors, March 22–23, 1965, New York, USOCLA, p. 82.

65. Minutes of the USOC Board of Directors, May 8, 1965, [no location given], USOCLA, p. 98.

66. Minutes of the USOC Board of Directors, October 25–26, New York, USOCLA, p. 66.

67. Proposal signed by Marquess of Exeter, Avery Brundage Collection, Box 82, 1966, Folder "Proposal by Marquess of Exeter: Training at High Altitudes, 1966."

68. Agenda of the Meeting of the IOC Medical Commission, December 20, 1967, Lausanne, quoted in Wrynn, "The Human Factor," 221. There was, it should be mentioned, one exception to this generalization: a February 1967 article by medical commission member Albert Dirix addressed high-altitude physiology. Albert Dirix, "The Problems of Altitude and Doping in Mexico," *Bulletin du Comité International Olympique*, February 1967, 43–46.

69. "Acclimatization at the Mexico Altitude," Minutes of the IOC General Session, April 1966, Rome, Annex 4, IOCL.

70. Minutes of the USOC Board of Directors, May 22, 1966, Washington, DC, USOCLA, p. 153.

71. Minutes of the USOC Board of Directors, February, 25–26, 1967, Chicago, USOCLA, pp. 235–236.

72. Roland Huntford, "Olympic Training: Inside Russia's Non-existent Camp," *Observer* (London), April 9, 1967. Clipping found in Avery Brundage Collection, Box 177, Folder "Games of XIX Olympiad—Mexico—Medical Board—Altitude, etc., 1964–68." On Soviet high-altitude camps, see also "Soviet Olympic Body in Study," *New York Times,* March 13, 1965; Wrynn, "'A Debt Was Paid Off in Tears,'" 1159.

73. "Training Camps," Circular Letter to the National Olympic Committees, August 11, 1967, quoted in Wrynn, "'A Debt Was Paid Off in Tears,'" 1164.

74. Dooley quoted in Bil Gilbert, "Drugs in Sport: Problems in a Turned On World," 66, 68.

75. Jack Scott, "It's Not How You Play the Game, But What Pill You Take," *New York Times,* October 17, 1971; Scott, "Drugs in Sports," *Chicago Tribune,* October 24, 1971; Todd, "A History of the Use of Anabolic Steroids in Sport," 327; Todd and Todd, "Significant Events in the History of Drug Testing and the Olympic Movement," 69.

76. See Todd, "Anabolic Steroids," 95.

77. Ibid.

78. Not surprisingly, when the IOC finally created a list of banned drugs in 1967, cannabis was included, even though no one could argue that it was a performance enhancer. See Minutes of the IOC General Session, May 3–9, 1967, Tehran, IOCL, Annex XIa. It should be mentioned, though, that cannabis was not included on the IOC's list of substances that would be tested for at the 1968 Winter Olympics in Grenoble. See "Medical Commission," *[IOC] Newsletter* (February 1968), 71.

79. Hubert H. Humphrey, "Senator Humphrey Appeals to Rival U.S. Sports Groups to End Feud over 1964 Olympics: Asks State Department [for] Report on Soviet Use of Athletes in 'Cold War'," September 10, 1962, File 14, Box 92, Series 3, Group II, Bureau of Educational and Cultural Affairs Historical Collection, University of Arkansas, Fayetteville, Arkansas (hereafter CU).

80. Hubert H. Humphrey, untitled document, n.d., Folder 14, Box 92, Series 3, Group II, CU.

81. Minutes of the IOC Executive Board, July 9–10, 1965, Paris, IOCL, p. 4.

82. Minutes of the IOC General Session, October 1965, Madrid, IOCL, p. 18.

83. Minutes of the IOC General Session, April 1966, Rome, IOCL, p. 3.

84. Minutes of the IOC General Session, April 1966, Rome, IOCL, Annex no. 11, p. 21. The report on doping, dated March 3, 1966, is contained in this annex. It is also available in Avery Brundage Collection, Box 82, Folder "RS Report by Committee on Doping, 1966."

85. See Wrynn, "The Human Factor," 220.

86. J. W. Westerhoff to Porritt, March 7, 1967, Avery Brundage Collection, Box 99, Folder "SP Medical Commission, IOC, 1966–1969."

87. Minutes of the IOC Executive Board, October 22, 1966, Mexico City, IOCL, p. 11.

88. Porritt to Avery Brundage, November 8, 1966, Avery Brundage Collection, Box 99, Folder "SP Medical Commission, IOC, 1966–1969."

89. Minutes of the IOC Executive Board, October 22, 1966, Mexico City, IOCL, p. 11.

90. Minutes of the IOC General Session, May 1967, Tehran, IOCL, p. 13.

91. Emphasis in original. This quote (p. 151) as well as the biographical information upon which this paragraph is based, come from David Miller, *Olympic Revolution: The Biography of Juan Antonio Samaranch,* rev. ed. (London: Pavilion, 1996).

92. De Merode's disagreement with powerful sanctions was present throughout his long tenure as medical commission chair. Even after Canadian sprinter Ben Johnson's positive test for steroids at the 1988 Seoul Olympic Games, for example, de Merode opposed lifetime suspensions. At a 1989 IOC general session, de Merode said that he was "strongly opposed to a 'life sentence'" for doping offenses. Minutes of the IOC General Session, August 30–September 1, 1989, San Juan, Puerto Rico, p. 12, copy on file at the Todd-McLean Physical Culture Collection, H. J. Lutcher Stark Center for Physical Culture and Sport, University of Texas at Austin.

93. Minutes of the IOC General Session, May 1967, Tehran, Annex XIa: "Doping"; Annex XIb: "Summary on Anabolic Steroids" (dated September 23, 1966), IOCL.

94. J. W. Westerhoff to Eduardo Hay, August 30, 1967, Avery Brundage Collection, Box 177, Folder "Games of XIX Olympiad—Mexico—Medical Board—Altitude, etc., 1964–68."

95. Todd and Todd, "Significant Events in the History of Drug Testing and the Olympic Movement," 67. Chaired by Prince Alexandre de Merode, the medical commission included eight other members, seven of whom were physicians or scientists: Arpad Csanadi (who, like de Merode, was not a medical expert), Dr. Albert Dirix, Dr. Arnold Beckett, Dr. Roger Genin, Professor Ludwig Prokop, Dr. Eduardo Hay, Dr. Pieter Van Dijk, and Professor Giuseppe La Cava. Press Release, IOC Medical Commission, September 27, 1967, Avery Brundage Collection, Box 99, Folder "SP Medical Commission, IOC, 1966–69."

96. Press Release, IOC Medical Commission, September 27, 1967.

CHAPTER 2

1. Emphasis in the original. Minutes of the IOC Medical Commission, December 20, 1967, Lausanne, Avery Brundage Collection, Box 99, Folder "SP Medical Commission, IOC, 1966–69," pp. 1–3.

2. K. S. "Sandy" Duncan to Avery Brundage, December 27, 1967, Avery Brundage Collection, Box 99, Folder "SP Medical Commission, IOC, 1966–69."

3. Ibid.

4. Daniel Hanley to Prince Alexandre de Merode, November 1, 1967, Robert Kane Papers, Box 4-a, Folder 4, USOCLA.

5. Pedro Ramirez Vásquez to Avery Brundage, July 21, 1967, Avery Brundage Collection, Box 177, Folder "Games of XIX Olympiad—Mexico—Medical Board—Altitude, etc., 1964–68."

6. J. W. Westerhoff to International Sports Federations, October 31, 1967, Avery Brundage Collection, Box 71, Folder [illegible].

7. Minutes of the IOC Executive Board, January 26–27, 1968, in Lausanne, and January 29–30, 1968, in Grenoble, IOCL, Annex III.

8. Minutes of the IOC General Session, January–February 1972, Sapporo, IOCL, p. 28.

9. Minutes of the IOC General Session, February 1968, Grenoble, IOCL, Annex II-a, pp. 3, 19.

10. Brundage to Prince Alexandre de Merode and Members of the IOC Executive Board, August 29, 1968, Avery Brundage Collection, Box 99, Folder "SP Medical Commission, IOC, 1966–69," p. 17.

11. Report by Doctor Thiebault on the Grenoble Games, n.d., Avery Brundage Collection, Box 99, Folder "SP Medical Commission, IOC, 1966–69," p. 17.

12. Minutes of the IOC Executive Board, September 1968, Mexico City, IOCL, p. 6.

13. For a short description of this pairing, see C. L. Cole, "Testing for Sex or Drugs," *Journal of Sport and Social Issues* 24, no. 4 (November 2000): 331–333. On sex testing during the 1960s at the Olympics, see also Wrynn, "The Human Factor," 221–224; Louis J. Elasas et al., "Gender Verification of Female Athletes," *Genetics in Medicine* 2, no. 4 (July–August 2000): 250.

14. Elasas et al., "Gender Verification of Female Athletes," 250. The fixation among Western officials with Eastern-bloc gender cheating is documented in Stefan Wiederkehr, "'We Shall Never Know the Exact Number of Men Who Have Competed in the Olympics Posing as Women': Sport, Gender Verification and the Cold War," *International Journal of the History of Sport* 26, no. 4 (March 2009): 556–572.

15. Marie-Thérèse Eyquem, "Women, Sports, and the Olympic Games," *Bulletin du Comité International Olympique,* February 1961, 50. On this point, see also Wrynn, "The Human Factor," 217.

16. Monique Berlioux, "Femininity," *Lettre d'information/Newsletter/Carta información,* December 1967, 1.

17. Minutes of the IOC Executive Board, October 22, 1966, Mexico City, IOCL, p. 11.

18. Brundage to Porritt, November 1, 1966, Avery Brundage Collection, Box 99, Folder "SP Medical Commission, IOC, 1966–1969."

19. Porritt to Brundage, November 8, 1966, Avery Brundage Collection, Box 99, Folder "SP Medical Commission, IOC, 1966–1969."

20. Michael Morris Killanin, *My Olympic Years* (New York: William Morrow, 1983), 157.

21. Minutes of the IOC General Session, May 1967, Tehran, IOCL, p. 13.

22. Minutes of the IOC Medical Commission, December 20, 1967, Lausanne, Avery Brundage Collection, Box 99, Folder "SP Medical Commission, IOC, 1966–1969," p. 4.

23. Daniel Hanley to Prince Alexandre de Merode, November 1, 1967, Robert Kane Papers, Box 4-a, Folder 4, USOCLA.

24. Minutes of the IOC Medical Commission, December 20, 1967, Lausanne, Avery Brundage Collection, Box 99, Folder "SP Medical Commission, IOC, 1966–1969," p. 4.

25. Minutes of the IOC Executive Board, January 26–27, 1968, in Lausanne, and January 29–30, 1968, in Grenoble, IOCL, Annex III, p. 2.

26. Individuals with XX chromosome patterns are defined as females. Those with XY patterns are defined as males. There are, however, exceptions to this generalization.

A number of medical conditions exist in which individuals can be genetically male or female while having the physical characteristics of the opposite gender. One out of approximately 500 to 600 female athletes, for instance, are affected by androgen insensitivity syndrome. While these women have the chromosomal characteristics of men, the inability of their tissue to be affected by androgens means that they develop female physical characteristics. See J. Stephenson, "Female Olympians' Sex Tests Outmoded," *Journal of the American Medical Association* 276, no. 3 (July 17, 1996): 177–178.

27. Minutes of the IOC General Session, February 1968, Grenoble, IOCL, Annex IIa.

28. Report by Doctor Thiebault on the Grenoble Games, n.d., Avery Brundage Collection, Box 99, Folder "SP Medical Commission, IOC, 1966–69," pp. 1–2.

29. Ibid., p. 1 (emphasis added).

30. Ibid.

31. Avery Brundage to General José de J. Clark, August 9, 1968, Avery Brundage Collection, Box 99, Folder "SP Medical Commission, IOC, 1966–69."

32. Emphasis in original. Avery Brundage to Prince Alexandre de Merode, August [illegible], 1968, Avery Brundage Collection, Box 99, Folder "SP Medical Commission, IOC, 1966–69."

33. Brundage to Prince Alexandre de Merode and members of the IOC Executive Board, August 29, 1968, Avery Brundage Collection, Box 99, Folder "SP Medical Commission, IOC, 1966–69."

34. Brundage Circular Letter to International Federations, National Olympic Committees, and International Olympic Committee, August 27, 1968, Avery Brundage Collection, Box 71, Folder "Circular Letters to IOC's, NOC's, IF's, 1968."

35. Prince Alexandre de Merode to IOC members, IOC Executive Board, and members of the Medical Commission, September 10, 1968, Avery Brundage Collection, Box 99, Folder "SP Medical Commission, IOC, 1966–69." This document can also be found in Avery Brundage Collection, Box 177, Folder "Games of XIX Olympiad—Mexico—Medical Board—Altitude, etc., 1964–1968."

36. José de J. Clark to Brundage, September 2, 1968, Avery Brundage Collection, Box 99, Folder "SP Medical Commission, IOC, 1966–69."

37. Brundage to Vásquez, August 31, 1968, Avery Brundage Collection, Box 177, Folder "Games of XIX Olympiad—Mexico—Medical Board—Altitude, etc., 1964–1968."

38. Brundage cablegram to de Merode, September 14, 1968, Avery Brundage Collection, Box 177, Folder "Games of XIX Olympiad—Mexico—Medical Board—Altitude, etc., 1964–1968."

39. Brundage to de Merode, September 14, 1968, Avery Brundage Collection, Box 71, Folder "Circular Letters to IOC's, NOC's, IF, 1968."

40. Telegram received by Brundage, marked "received" on September 16, 1968, Avery Brundage Collection, Box 99, Folder "SP Medical Commission, IOC, 1966–69."

41. De Merode to Brundage, September 24, 1968, Avery Brundage Collection, Box 71, Folder "Circular Letters to IOC's, NOC's, IF's, 1968."

42. Brundage and de Merode cited from Minutes of the IOC Executive Board, September 30, 1968–October 6, 1968, Mexico City, IOCL, p. 6. Brundage repeated the explanation for his stance at a later (October 7–11, 1968) IOC general session in Mexico City. See page 12 of the minutes of that session, which are also available at the IOCL.

43. "General Report Presented by Dr. Eduardo Hay, Member of the Medical Commission of the International Olympic Committee and Delegate of the Organizing Committee of the Games of the XIX Olympiad—Mexico, October 1968," IOC Medical Commission Series, Folder "Commission Médicale: Rapports de Grenoble et de Mexico, 1968 à 1969," IOCL, pp. 2–5. A copy of this essential document is also contained in Avery Brundage Collection, Box 99, Folder "SP Medical Commission, IOC, 1966–69."

44. "General Report Presented by Dr. Eduardo Hay," pp. 5–14. This set of procedures is detailed in A. H. Beckett, G. T. Tucker, and A. C. Moffat, "Routine Detection and Identification in Urine of Stimulants and Other Drugs, Some of Which May Be Used to Modify Performance in Sport," *Journal of Pharmacy and Pharmacology* 19, no. 5 (May 1967): 273–294.

45. The positive tests were reported in "General Report Presented by Dr. Eduardo Hay," pp. 12–13. Hay is quoted on page 15.

46. Quoted in Gilbert, "Drugs in Sport: Problems in a Turned On World," 66.

47. "General Report Presented by Dr. Eduardo Hay," p. 15.

48. Quoted in Gilbert, "Drugs in Sport: Problems in a Turned On World," 66.

49. For Americans' interpretation of athletics as a "pure" exception to everyday life, see Michael Mandelbaum, *The Meaning of Sports: Why Americans Watch Baseball, Football, and Basketball, and What They See When They Do* (New York: Public Affairs, 2004), 4–9.

50. Gilbert, "Drugs in Sport: Problems in a Turned On World," 64.

CHAPTER 3

1. For an insightful interpretation of Olympic internationalism, see John M. Hoberman, "Toward a Theory of Olympic Internationalism," *Journal of Sport History* 22, no. 1 (Spring 1995): 1–37. See also Hoberman, *The Olympic Crisis: Sport, Politics, and the Moral Order* (New Rochelle, NY: A. D. Caratzas, 1986). A wonderful recent analysis of the tension between nationalism and internationalism in athletics prior to the Second World War is provided in Keys, *Globalizing Sport*. See also Keys, "The Internationalization of Sport, 1890–1939," in *The Cultural Turn: Essays in the History of U.S. Foreign Relations,* ed. Frank A. Ninkovich and Liping Bu (Chicago: Imprint Publications, 2001), 201–220; Keys, "Spreading Peace, Democracy, and Coca-Cola: Sport and American Cultural Expansion in the 1930s," *Diplomatic History* 28, no. 2 (April 2004): 165–196.

2. "Sincere" internationalism was Coubertin's term for this environment. See William J. Morgan, "Cosmopolitanism, Olympism, and Nationalism: A Critical Interpretation of Coubertin's Ideal of International Sporting Life," *Olympika: The International Journal of Olympic Studies* 4 (1995): 81. De Coubertin's assertion that nationalism was "by no means detrimental" is quoted on page 88.

3. Coubertin quoted in Hoberman, *The Olympic Crisis,* 51. Coubertin also asserted that in the wake of the First World War "ulterior motives of a nationalistic or a religious character . . . would only upset the whole [Olympic] movement in the end." Pierre de Coubertin, *Olympic Memoirs* (Lausanne: International Olympic Committee, 1997), 185. The best biography of Coubertin is John J. MacAloon, *This Great Symbol:*

Pierre de Coubertin and the Origins of the Modern Olympic Games (Chicago: University of Chicago Press, 1981).

4. Minutes of the IOC General Session, May 1970, Amsterdam, IOCL, p. 112.

5. "Report of the Chairman of the Medical Commission of the International Olympic Committee," September 1971, Luxemburg, IOC Medical Commission Records, Box SD 1: Comm. Méd.: Rapp. Sessions, CE 1968–1984, IOCL.

6. For the GDR's doping program, see Steven Ungerleider, *Faust's Gold: Inside the East German Doping Machine* (New York: Thomas Dunne Books / St. Martin's Press, 2001); Brigitte Berendonk, *Doping Dokumente: Von der Forschung zum Betrug* (Berlin: Springer-Verlag, 1991); Werner W. Franke and Brigitte Berendonk, "Hormonal Doping and Androgenization of Athletes: A Secret Program of the German Democratic Republic Government," *Clinical Chemistry* 43, no. 7 (July 1997): 1262–1279; Giselher Spitzer, "A Leninist Monster: Compulsory Doping and Public Policy in the G.D.R. and the Lessons for Today," in *Doping and Public Policy,* ed. John M. Hoberman and Verner Møller (Odense: University Press of Southern Denmark, 2004), 133–143. An early, sympathetic analysis of the East German sport system is provided in Doug Gilbert, *The Miracle Machine* (New York: Coward, McCann, & Geoghegan, 1980).

7. George Orwell, "The Sporting Spirit," *Tribune* (London), December 14, 1945. See also Philip Goodhart and Christopher Chataway, *War without Weapons* (London: W. H. Allen, 1968). For a collection of monographs on the relationship of militarism to sport, see the special edition (vol. 5, June 2003) of the *European Sport History Review,* "Militarism, Sport, Europe: War without Weapons."

8. Minutes of the IOC Executive Board, March 22–23, 1969, Lausanne, IOCL, p. 6.

9. Ibid., p. 7.

10. Minutes of the IOC Executive Board, June 5–9, 1969, Warsaw, IOCL, p. 5.

11. Brundage to de Merode, May 2, 1971, Avery Brundage Collection, Box 99, Folder "Medical Commission, 1970–73."

12. Berlioux to Brundage, March 24, 1971, Avery Brundage Collection, Box 99, Folder "Medical Commission, 1970–73"; Brundage to Berlioux, April 20, 1971, Avery Brundage Collection, Box 99, Folder "Medical Commission, 1970–73."

13. Brundage to de Merode, April 22, 1971, Avery Brundage Collection, Box 99, Folder "Medical Commission, 1970–73."

14. Minutes of the Meeting of the Working Group of the IOC Medical Commission, July 29, 1971, Avery Brundage Collection, Folder "Medical Commission, 1970–73"; de Merode remarks in IOC General Session, Luxemburg, September 11–18, 1971, IOCL, Annex 17, p. 33.

15. IOC brochure, "Doping," Lausanne, 1972, IOC Medical Commission Records, Folder "Commission Médicale: Correspondence et cas de dopage, 1972 à 1973," IOCL, p. 4.

16. Minutes of the IOC Medical Commission, Sapporo, January 29–30, and February 3, 1972, Avery Brundage Collection, Box 99, Folder "Medical Commission, 1970–73."

17. Brundage to de Merode, November 1, 1971, Avery Brundage Collection, Box 99, Folder "Medical Commission, 1970–73"; Report of the Medical Commission, IOC General Session, Luxemburg, September 11–18, 1971, IOCL, p. 23.

18. Report of the Medical Commission, IOC General Session, Luxemburg, September 11–18, 1971, IOCL, p. 23.

19. Minutes of the IOC Executive Board, March 22–23, 1969, Lausanne, IOCL, p. 6.

20. Report of the Medical Commission, IOC General Session, Luxemburg, September 11–18, 1971, IOCL, p. 23.

21. Proposal of the Belgian Olympic Committee, Minutes of the IOC Executive Board, May 27–30, 1972, Lausanne, IOCL, p. 13.

22. Minutes of the Meeting of the USOC Board of Directors, October 11–12, 1971, New York, USOCLA, p. 92.

23. U.S. Senate, Committee on the Judiciary, Subcommittee to Investigate Juvenile Delinquency, *Hearings Pursuant to S. Res. 56, Section 12. Investigative Hearings on the Proper and Improper Use of Drugs by Athletes,* 93rd Congress, 1st sess., June 18, July 12, 13, 1973 (Washington, DC: U.S. Government Printing Office, 1973), 274.

24. Patera quoted in Scott, "It's Not How You Play the Game, but What Pill You Take."

25. Terry Todd telephone interview with Ken Patera, May 16, 1986, quoted in Todd, "Anabolic Steroids," 95.

26. Minutes of the Meeting of the USOC Board of Directors, October 11–12, 1971, New York, USOCLA, p. 89.

27. Todd and Todd, "Significant Events in the History of Drug Testing and the Olympic Movement: 1960–1999," 70. Schloder was identified in IOC Press Release, February 11, 1972, Sapporo, IOC Medical Commission Records, Folder "Dopage aux Jeux Olympiques d'Hiver de Sapporo 1972: Rapports d'analyse, résultets et correspondence," 1972, IOCL.

28. IOC brochure, "Doping," Lausanne, 1972, IOC Medical Commission Records, Folder "Commission Médicale: Correspondence et cas de dopage, 1972 à 1973," IOCL, p. 45.

29. Minutes of the IOC General Session, August 21–24, September 5, 1972, Munich, IOCL, p. 32.

30. Erik Strömgren, Johannes Nielsen, Mogens Ingerslov, Gert Bruun Petersen, and A. J. Therkelsen, "A Memorandum on the Use of Sex Chromatin Investigation of Competitors in Women's Divisions of the Olympic Games," February 3, 1972, Avery Brundage Collection, Box 99, Folder "Medical Commission, 1970–73."

31. "Those Exempted Have 'Passes'," *Los Angeles Times,* January 17, 1972.

32. Erik Strömgren et al., "A Memorandum on the Use of Sex Chromatin Investigation of Competitors in Women's Divisions of the Olympic Games," February 3, 1972, Avery Brundage Collection, Box 99, Folder "Medical Commission, 1970–73."

33. Brundage to de Merode, April 24, 1972, Avery Brundage Collection, Box 99, Folder "Medical Commission, 1970–73."

34. Albert de la Chapelle, "The Use and Misuse of Sex Chromatin Screening for 'Gender Identification' of Female Athletes," *Journal of the American Medical Association* 256, no. 14 (October 10, 1986): 1920–1923.

35. At the Albertville Games, the IOC replaced chromatin tests with testing for "Y-specific loci using polymerase chain reaction (PCR) amplification of DNA extracted from nucleated buccal cells." Louis J. Elasas et al., "Gender Verification of Female Athletes," *Genetics in Medicine* 2, no. 4 (July–August 2000): 251.

36. De Merode and Brundage statements in Report of the Medical Commission, Minutes of the IOC Executive Board, May 27–30, 1972, Lausanne, IOCL, p. 28.

37. Report of the Munich Organizing Committee, IOC General Session, January–February 1972, Sapporo, IOCL, Annex 5, pp. 56–57.

38. Dr. R. Marlier, "Report of the Medical Commission of the 'International Cycling Union'," January 13, 1968, attached to Artur Takac [IOC technical director] to Suat Erler [secretary general, Turkish Olympic Committee], September 24, 1971, IOC Medical Commission Records, Box SD 1: Comm. Méd.: Rapp. Sessions, CE 1968–1984, IOCL.

39. Todd, "A History of the Use of Anabolic Steroids in Sport," 330.

40. O'Shea quoted in "Team Physiologist Claims Nearly All U.S. Weightlifters on Steroids," *Los Angeles Times*, July 16, 1972. This article mistakenly identified Pat O'Shea as Pat O'Rea.

41. Zeigler quoted in "Team Physiologist Claims Nearly All U.S. Weightlifters on Steroids."

42. See Sharon Robb, "Burned: At the Munich Olympics of 1972, a Young Swimmer Named Rick DeMont Was Stripped of His Gold Medal Due to a Bureaucratic Error. Think That Sounds like an Easy Fix? Not Even Close," *Splash: The Official Newsletter of United States Swimming*, April–May 2001, 8–9.

43. DeMont to de Merode, September 4, 1972, Avery Brundage Collection, Box 185, Folder "XXth Olympiad, Status of Rick DeMont's Gold Medal."

44. Winston P. Rhiel to Alexandre de Merode, September 3, 1972, IOC Medical Commission Records, Folder "Cas de dopage: PV organization du contrôle de dopage athlétisme, basketball, boxe, cyclisme, etc., 1972 à 1972," IOCL. Given the continuing need to refine definitions of doping, it should be noted that recent scientific studies question the notion that asthma medications boost athletic performance. See Gina Kolata, "Asthma Medications: Not a Clear Advantage," *New York Times*, July 22, 2008.

45. Clifford H. Buck to de Merode, September 4, 1972, Avery Brundage Collection, Box 185, Folder "XXth Olympiad, Status of Rick DeMont's Gold Medal."

46. De Merode's initial advocation that DeMont keep his medal is contained in Minutes of the IOC Executive Board, August 18–22 and September 1, 6–8, 10–11, 1972, IOCL, p. 41. The medical commission's subsequent position is outlined in both these minutes and a letter: de Merode to Brundage, September 4, 1972, IOC Medical Commission Records, Folder "Cas de dopage: PV organization du contrôle de dopage athlétisme, basketball, boxe, cyclisme, etc., 1972 à 1972," IOCL. De Merode's statements in this paragraph are quoted from the letter.

47. Brundage to Clifford Buck, September 8, 1972, IOC Medical Commission Records, Folder "Dopage: Rick DeMont (USA Swimming) et Patrick James (American Basketball Team), etc., 1972 à 1973," IOCL. The executive board's decision regarding DeMont is provided in Minutes of the IOC Executive Board, August 18–22 and September 1, 6–8, 10–11, 1972, IOCL, p. 47. The USOC's account of the events surrounding DeMont's punishment is provided in "The Rick DeMont 'Doping' Charge," September 29, 1972, appended to Proceedings of the Executive Committee of the Board of Directors of the United States Olympic Committee, November 6, 1972, USOCLA.

48. For a contemporaneous observation of the U.S. perceptions of an anti-American prejudice among Olympic leaders in Munich, see Richard D. Mandell, *A Munich Diary: The Olympics of 1972* (Chapel Hill: University of North Carolina Press, 1991), 168.

49. For the communiqué and its description, see Mandell, *A Munich Diary*, 147–148.

50. Memorandum, "Subject: Modern Pentathlon Doping Procedures at XX Olympiad," IOC Medical Commission Records, Folder "Cas de dopage: PV organization du contrôle de dopage athlétisme, basketball, boxe, cyclisme, etc., 1972 à 1972," IOCL.

51. Press Release from the IOC Medical Commission, September 8, 1972, IOC Medical Commission Records, Folder "Cas de dopage: PV organization du contrôle de dopage athlétisme, basketball, boxe, cyclisme, etc., 1972 à 1972," IOCL.

52. Press Release from the IOC Medical Commission, September 8, 1972, IOC Medical Commission Records, Folder "Cas de dopage: PV organization du contrôle de dopage athlétisme, basketball, boxe, cyclisme, etc., 1972 à 1972," IOCL.

53. Wille Grut to Dieter Krickow, n.d.; Krickow, "To the Members of the International Jury, Delegation Heads, and Team Captains of Participating Teams. Subject: Doping Control on the Occasion of the Olympic Modern Pentathlon Competition," August 24, 1972. Both documents are from IOC Medical Commission Records, Folder "Cas de dopage: PV organization du contrôle de dopage athlétisme, basketball, boxe, cyclisme, etc., 1972 à 1972," IOCL.

54. The Munich newspaper *BILD* ran a story on September 3, 1972, indicating sixteen positive results. The next day, *BILD* identified sixteen Olympians from Finland, Sweden, Holland, and Austria. A clipping of the September 3 story and translations of both can be found in Tab F of Memorandum, "Subject: Modern Pentathlon Doping Procedures at XX Olympiad."

55. Minutes of the IOC Executive Board, August 18–22 and September 1, 6–8, 10–11, 1972, IOCL, p. 40.

56. Evidence presented in Minutes of the IOC Executive Board, August 18–22 and September 1, 6–8, 10–11, 1972, IOCL, p. 40. Grut quoted in Grut to IOC Medical Commission, The Chairman, September 2, 1972, IOC Medical Commission Records, Folder "Cas de dopage: PV organization du contrôle de dopage athlétisme, basketball, boxe, cyclisme, etc., 1972 à 1972," IOCL.

57. Brundage to de Merode, October 5, 1972, Avery Brundage Collection, Box 99, Folder "Medical Commission, 1970–73"; Press Release signed by de Merode, n.d., Avery Brundage Collection, Box 99, Folder "Medical Commission, 1970–73."

58. Buck to Lord Killanin, September 27, 1972, IOC Medical Commission Records, Folder "Cas de dopage: PV organization du contrôle de dopage athlétisme, basketball, boxe, cyclisme, etc., 1972 à 1972," IOCL.

59. Minutes of the IOC Executive Board, August 18–22 and September 1, 6–8, 10–11, 1972, IOCL, p. 46.

60. Ibid., pp. 41–47. The response from the national Olympic committee of The Netherlands is provided in Annex 14 of these minutes. Jones's statement can be found on p. 43.

CHAPTER 4

1. See Miller, *Olympic Revolution*, 11.
2. Coupat quoted in Miller, *Olympic Revolution*, 11.

3. Minutes of the IOC Executive Board, February 2–5, 1973, Lausanne, IOCL, p. 12.

4. General Hains quoted in Proceedings of the Meeting of the USOC Board of Directors, January 3–4, 1973, USOCLA, p. 232.

5. U.S. Senate, *Investigative Hearings on the Proper and Improper Use of Drugs by Athletes,* 150.

6. James quoted in Neil Amdur, "Use of Caffeine Cited: Drugs Played an Olympic Role," *International Herald Tribune,* November 15, 1972.

7. U.S. Senate, *Investigative Hearings on the Proper and Improper Use of Drugs by Athletes,* 151.

8. This regulation was successfully proposed by Lord Killanin in Minutes of the IOC Executive Board, February 2–5, 1973, Lausanne, IOCL. For the connection between American protests and the decision to bar team physicians from membership on the IOC medical commission, see Minutes of the IOC Executive Board, September 29–30 and October 2, 1973, IOCL, p. 28. In that document, de Merode stated, "The experience in Munich of the team doctor attached to the US team was sufficient evidence of this" need for "the decision that doctors of teams at the Olympic Games should not be members of the Medical Commission."

9. On the use of sport to produce a sense of East German nationhood among GDR citizens, consult Tara Magdalinski, "Sports History and East German National Identity," *Peace Review* 11, no. 4 (December 1999): 539–545. Though it concentrates on the 1950s, see for a larger analysis Molly Wilkinson Johnson, *Training Socialist Citizens: Sports and the State in East Germany* (Boston: Brill, 2008).

10. Article 18 of the East German Constitution provided, "Physical culture, sport and outdoor pursuits promote, as elements of socialist culture, the all-round physical and mental development of the individual." Quoted in Günter Witt, "Mass Participation and Top Performance in One: Physical Culture and Sport in the German Democratic Republic," *Journal of Popular Culture* 18, no. 3 (Winter 1984): 171.

11. Cha, *Beyond the Final Score,* 21. In terms of specific numbers, Cha writes that "the East Germans won one gold medal for every 425,000 citizens (versus the United States at one gold per 6.5 million citizens)."

12. Richard W. Pound, *Inside Dope,* 54.

13. Witness Deposition of Henrich Misersky in the Civil Suit Kurt Hinze v. Jens Steinigen, Case # 9081/91, n.d., District Court of Mainz, Box 2X89, CD 1, Steven Ungerleider Collection, Dolph Briscoe Center for American History, University of Texas at Austin (translated copy; original in German).

14. For a wide-ranging, nuanced analysis of the early East German–Soviet relationship, consult Hope M. Harrison, *Driving the Soviets Up the Wall: Soviet–East German Relations, 1953–1963* (Princeton, NJ: Princeton University Press, 2003).

15. Ladislav Pataki and Lee Holden, *Winning Secrets: Confessions of a Soviet Bloc Sports Scientist* (n.p.: Training Management Systems: 1989), 166–167.

16. See Franke and Berendonk, "Hormonal Doping and Androgenization of Athletes," 1264.

17. Quoted in Ungerleider, *Faust's Gold,* 146.

18. The medal count for the Games is provided on the IOC website, www.olympics.org.

19. Ungerleider, *Faust's Gold,* 88.

20. Quoted in Franke and Berendonk, "Hormonal Doping and Androgenization of Athletes," 1264.

21. Ungerleider, *Faust's Gold*, 107.

22. Minutes of the IOC Executive Board, February 2–5, 1973, IOCL, pp. 12–13.

23. Minutes of the IOC Executive Board, September 29–39 and October 2, 1973, IOCL, p. 14.

24. "Prince de Merode's Report to the Session—May 1975," IOC Medical Commission Documents, Folder "SD 1: Comm. Méd.: Rapp. Sessions, CE 1968–1984," IOCL.

25. R. V. Brooks, R. G. Firth, and N. A. Sumner, "Detection of Anabolic Steroids by Radioimmunoassay," *British Journal of Sports Medicine* 9, no. 2 (July 1975): 89–92; R. J. Ward, C. H. Shackleton, and A. M. Lawson, "Gas Chromatographic-Mass Spectrometric Methods for the Detection and Identification of Anabolic Steroid Drugs," *British Journal of Sports Medicine* 9, no. 2 (July 1975): 93–97. See also Todd, "A History of the Use of Anabolic Steroids in Sport," 330.

26. The IOC announced steroid tests for the 1976 Montreal Games in Minutes of the IOC General Session, October 21–24, 1974, Vienna, IOCL, p. 19. For the way in which the two procedures were used, see A. H. Beckett, "Misuse of Drugs in Sport," *British Journal of Sports Medicine* 12 (January 1979): 189.

27. See Beckett, "Misuse of Drugs in Sport," 191.

28. Lord Killanin quoted in "British Find Method to Detect Steroids," *Los Angeles Times*, November 1, 1973.

29. See Beckett, "Misuse of Drugs in Sport," 191.

30. Bannister quoted in "British Find Method to Detect Steroids."

31. Dr. Manfred Donike (later head of the IOC drug-testing committee), personal communication to Terry Todd, April 1987, referenced in Todd, "A History of the Use of Anabolic Steroids in Sport," 330. At a May 1975 IOC executive board meeting, James Worrall, a member of the Montreal organizing committee's board of directors, noted that "the control of anabolic steroids [at the Montreal Games] would be difficult on account of the cost." Quoted in Minutes of the IOC Executive Board, May 14–16, 1975, Rome, and May 19, 23, 1975, Lausanne, IOCL, p. 26.

32. Minutes of the IOC General Session, October 21–24, 1974, Vienna, IOCL, p. 19.

33. See "Steroid Drug Tests to Be Held," *Chicago Tribune*, September 1, 1974.

34. Ibid.

35. "Steroids Are Out and Marks Are Down in Some Field Events," *Los Angeles Times*, September 9, 1974.

36. See Todd, "A History of the Use of Anabolic Steroids in Sport," 330.

37. "Anabolic Steroid Control," July 16, 1976, IOC Medical Commission Records, Folder "Dopage en haltérophilie aux Jeux Olympiques de Montréal 1976, 1976 à 1977," IOCL. The subcommittee members were Arnold H. Beckett, I. M. Diop, Robert Dugal, Michel Bertrand, and Albert Nantel. They are listed on page 4 of the aforementioned document.

38. This position had been put forward at an IOC meeting held the previous year. "The list of banned substances now included anabolic steroids, which were to be checked *before* the Games began" (emphasis in the original). Minutes of the IOC General Session, May 21–23, 1975, Lausanne, IOCL, p. 18.

39. "Anabolic Steroid Control," July 16, 1976, IOC Medical Commission Records, Folder "Dopage en haltérophilie aux Jeux Olympiques de Montréal 1976, 1976 à 1977," IOCL.

40. Ibid.

41. Minutes of the IOC General Session, July 13–17, 19, 1976, Montreal, IOCL, p. 41.

42. "Effect of Drugs to Aid Athletes Studied by U.S.," *New York Times,* August 22, 1976.

43. "Olympian Says Drug Use Heavy," *Chicago Tribune,* June 23, 1976.

44. These points can be found in Proceedings of the Meeting of the USOC Board of Directors, June 5, 1976, New York, USOCLA, pp. 99–114. Giegenbach quote from page 100.

45. Kenneth J. Bender and Dr. Dean H. Lockwood to Dr. Daniel F. Hanley, August 13, 1976, F. Don Miller Papers, Series IV, Box 41, Folder 442, USOCLA.

46. Beckett, "Misuse of Drugs in Sport," 190. For the ratio of anabolic steroid indications, see "Medical Report of the 1976 Montreal Olympic Games," IOC Medical Commission Records, Folder "SD 1: Comm. Méd.: Rapp. Sessions, CE 1968–1984," IOCL, pp. 10–11.

47. See "Cameron, Two Others Banned for Steroid Use," *Los Angeles Times,* July 31, 1976; Jerry Kirshenbaum, "Steroids: The Growing Menace," *Sports Illustrated,* November 12, 1979, 33.

48. "Games of the XXI Olympiad, Montreal, Canada, Bulletin," n.d., F. Don Miller Papers, Series IV, Box 41, Folder 442, USOCLA.

49. Ibid.

50. Kapitan to the President of the IOC [Killanin], September 3, 1976, IOC Medical Commission Records, Folder "Dopage en haltérophilie aux Jeux Olympiques de Montréal 1976, 1976 à 1977," IOCL.

51. Killanin to "Technical Director," August 31, 1976, IOC Medical Commission Records, Folder "Dopage en haltérophilie aux Jeux Olympiques de Montréal 1976, 1976 à 1977," IOCL.

52. Killanin to "Technical Director," September 1, 1976, IOC Medical Commission Records, Folder "Dopage en haltérophilie aux Jeux Olympiques de Montréal 1976, 1976 à 1977," IOCL.

53. "Weightlifting: New Tests Confirm Steroid Use by Five," *Times* (London), August 27, 1976, clipping in IOC Medical Commission Records, Folder "Dopage en haltérophilie aux Jeux Olympiques de Montréal 1976, 1976 à 1977," IOCL.

54. Untitled Medical Report, October 15, 1976, IOC Medical Commission Records, Folder "Dopage en haltérophilie aux Jeux Olympiques de Montréal 1976, 1976 à 1977," IOCL, p. 39.

55. Document 3 attached to "Report from Prof. Arnold H. Beckett, Member of the IOC Medical Commission on the Positive Cases of Anabolic Steroids, Announced after the Close of the 1976 Olympic Games at Montreal," signed by medical commission members Arnold H. Beckett, Daniel Hanley, and Carroll A. Laurin, August 23, 1976, IOC Medical Commission Records, Folder "Dopage en haltérophilie aux Jeux Olympiques de Montréal 1976, 1976 à 1977," IOCL.

56. Strachan is quoted in "E. German Women's Success Stirs U.S. Anger," *New York Times,* August 1, 1976.

57. White quoted in "E. German Women's Success Stirs U.S. Anger."

58. Dardik quoted in "Effect of Drugs to Aid Athletes Studied by U.S."

59. "Dr. Dardik's Sports Medicine Presentation," Athletes Advisory Council Meeting, Squaw Valley, California, April 2, 1977, appended as Exhibit "A" in Proceedings of the Quadrennial Meeting of the United States Olympic Committee, General Business Session, April 29, 1977, Colorado Springs, vol. 1, USOCLA.

60. White quoted in "Effect of Drugs to Aid Athletes Studied by U.S."

61. The effects of the GDR doping system for East German athletes are catalogued in Ungerleider, *Faust's Gold*.

62. Historians also quite naturally place greater emphasis on the Black September attacks than on doping issues in the context of the Munich Games. For example, doping was mentioned in only a handful of the 193 substantive pages of text in historian Richard D. Mandell's memoirs of the competitions: *A Munich Diary*, 162.

CHAPTER 5

1. The 1980 Moscow Games are covered in Christopher Booker, *The Games War: A Moscow Journal* (London: Faber and Faber, 1981); and Barukh Hazan, *Olympic Sports and Propaganda Games: Moscow 1980* (New Brunswick, NJ: Transaction Books, 1982). The boycott by an American-led coalition is analyzed in Hulme, *The Political Olympics*. The Soviet Union's retaliation with a similar boycott in 1984 has received less attention. For a starting point, see Harold E. Wilson, Jr., "The Golden Opportunity: Romania's Political Manipulation of the 1984 Los Angeles Olympic Games," *Olympika: The International Journal of Olympic Studies* 3 (1994): 83–97. An overview of the state of doping in sport at the beginning of the decade is provided in E. C. Percy, "Chemical Warfare: Drugs in Sports," *Western Journal of Medicine* 133, no. 6 (December 1980): 478–484.

2. "Purest" is the term used by IOC medical commission chair Alexandre de Merode. He is quoted in the Organising Committee for the 1980 Olympic Games in Moscow, "Doping Control at the Games of the XXIInd Olympiad," February 1981, IOC Medical Commission Records, Folder "Affaires Médicale aux Jeux Olympiques de Moscou 1980: Contrôles du dopage et de feminale 1980, 1980–1987," IOCL, p. 28.

3. For an interesting argument that economic incentives for effective doping controls should be implemented by sports authorities in order to counteract the current economic disincentives for their employment, see Wolfgang Maennig, "On the Economics of Doping and Corruption in International Sports," *Journal of Sports Economics* 3, no. 1 (February 2002): 61–89.

4. The 1980 Games illustrated the continuing weakness of Olympic doping policy, and the 1984 Los Angeles Games witnessed a doping "cover-up." Testosterone was finally added to the IOC's list of banned substances in 1982. See Todd and Todd, "Significant Events in the History of Drug Testing and the Olympic Movement," 78; and Philip Hage, "Caffeine, Testosterone Banned for Olympians," *Physician and Sportsmedicine* 10, no. 7 (July 1982): 15–17. The implications of the Johnson scandal for doping policy in international athletics are discussed in Judith Blackwell, "Discourses on Drug Use: The Social Construction of a Steroid Scandal," *Journal of Drug Issues* 21, no. 1 (Winter 1991): 147–164. See also Bruce Kidd, Robert Edelman, and Susan Brownell, "Comparative Analysis of Doping Scandals: Canada, Russia, and China," in

Doping in Elite Sport: The Politics of Drugs in the Olympic Movement, ed. Wayne Wilson and Edward Derse (Champaign, IL: Human Kinetics, 2001), 155–161.

5. Pound, *Inside the Olympics,* 53.

6. The interaction of private sports organizations and national governments on doping issues during the 1980s is briefly discussed in Houlihan, *Dying to Win,* 160.

7. Shorter quoted in "Effect of Drugs to Aid Athletes Studied by U.S."

8. Anderson quoted in Amdur, "Wider Olympic Drug Abuse Is Seen."

9. Rogozhin quoted in Barry Lorge, "IOC Gears Up to Detect Drugs, Ingenious Cheating in Moscow," *Washington Post,* June 1, 1979.

10. Hanley quoted in Lorge, "IOC Gears Up to Detect Drugs, Ingenious Cheating in Moscow."

11. See Ungerleider, *Faust's Gold,* 37–38. For a contemporaneous journalistic depiction, see Pete Axthelm and Frederick Kempe, "The East German Machine," *Newsweek,* July 14, 1980, 50.

12. Quoted in Lorge, "IOC Gears Up to Detect Drugs, Ingenious Cheating in Moscow."

13. Neufeld quoted in John Vinocur, "East German Tale of Tyranny," *New York Times,* January 11, 1979. Several other defectors from the GDR provided similar information. These included shot-putter Ilona Slupianek and Dr. Alois Marder, a former East German sports physician. See Michael Getler, "E. Germans, Drugs: Hard Facts Missing," *Washington Post,* May 27, 1979.

14. Vogel quoted in "Sporting Scene," *National Review* 31, no. 41 (October 12, 1979): 1280. Vogel also reported that she experienced medical problems because she had been subjected to compulsory doping since age fourteen.

15. The 1976 program is outlined in "Effect of Drugs to Aid Athletes Studied by U.S."

16. Miller quoted in Neil Amdur, "Mounting Drug Use Afflicts World Sports," *New York Times,* November 20, 1978.

17. Beckett quoted in Ken Denlinger, "Warfare on Drugs Increases," *Washington Post,* February 12, 1980.

18. Hess quoted in Paul Dimeo, "Saint or Sinner? A Reconsideration of the Career of Prince Alexandre de Merode, Chair of the International Olympic Committee's Medical Commission 1967–2002" (unpublished manuscript).

19. Dugal and Bertrand quoted in Steve Cady, "Drug Testers Stiffen Olympic Procedures," *New York Times,* December 7, 1979.

20. Daley quoted in Denlinger, "Warfare on Drugs Increases."

21. Beckett quoted in Denlinger, "Warfare on Drugs Increases."

22. There were 440 tests for stimulants and 350 tests for anabolic steroids. See "Olympic Athletes Cleared," *Washington Post,* February 25, 1980.

23. Berlioux quoted in Bill Starr, "Steroid Madness: Drugs and the Olympics," August 1980, p. 65, magazine clipping in IOC Medical Commission Records, Folder "Los Angeles '84 Medical Matters, 1978–1983," IOCL.

24. Andrew Nynka, "Ukrainian Scientist Details Secret Soviet Research Project on Steroids," *Ukrainian Weekly,* November 9, 2003, http://www.ukrweekly.com/Archive/2003/450319.shtml.

25. Medical Commission Report, Minutes of the IOC General Session, February 10–13, 1980, Lake Placid, IOCL, p. 24.

26. See Robert O. Voy and Kirk D. Deeter, *Drugs, Sport, and Politics: The Inside Story about Drug Use in Sport and Its Political Cover-up, with a Prescription for Reform* (Champaign, IL: Leisure Press, 1991), 112.

27. IOC medical commission member Dr. Arnold Beckett, observing the events in Moscow, said, "You see some of the shapes . . . and suspicions are probably justified." Beckett quoted in "I.O.C. Issues Doping Report," *New York Times*, August 4, 1980. A Russian sports journalist later laughingly told British journalist Andrew Jennings about the media's knowledge of the drug tests in Moscow: "'Doping control in Moscow? . . . There was no doping control!'" See Andrew Jennings, *The New Lords of the Rings* (London: Simon & Schuster, 1996), 236.

28. The numbers for the various drug tests in Moscow are provided in the Organising Committee for the 1980 Olympic Games in Moscow, "Doping Control at the Games of the XXIInd Olympiad," February 1981, IOC Medical Commission Records, Folder "Affaires Médicale aux Jeux Olympiques de Moscou 1980: Contrôles du dopage et de feminale 1980, 1980–1987," IOCL, p. 28.

29. Ibid.

30. Donike interview by Terry Todd, February 6, 1982, referenced in Todd and Todd, "Significant Events in the History of Drug Testing and the Olympic Movement," 77. See also Terry Todd, "A History of the Use of Anabolic Steroids in Sport," in *Sport and Exercise Science: Essays in the History of Sports Medicine*, ed. Jack W. Berryman and Roberta J. Park (Chicago: University of Illinois Press, 1992), 333.

31. Government of Australia, "Drugs in Sport," *Interim Report of the Senate Standing Committee on the Environment, Recreation and the Arts* (Canberra: Australian Government Publishing Service, 1989), p. 10, quoted in Houlihan, *Dying to Win*, 47.

32. The colonel also claimed that positive test results were suppressed for several Swedish and East German Olympians. See Jennings, *The New Lords of the Rings*, 235–236. According to a fellow English journalist, three Soviet security agents were appointed to the Soviet Olympic committee prior to the 1980 Games by KGB director Yuri Andropov. The KGB agents were Anatoly Gresko (who in 1971 had been thrown out of England for espionage), Semyon Nitkin (the controller for the notorious British double-agent Kim Philby), and V. I. Popov. See "Sporting Scene," 1280.

33. Minutes of the IOC General Session, Baden-Baden, September 29–October 2, 1981, IOCL, pp. 28–29.

34. Minutes of the IOC General Session, Baden-Baden, September 29–October 2, 1981, IOCL, p. 29.

35. Prince Alexandre de Merode, "Report from the IOC Medical Commission," Annex 13 of Minutes of the IOC General Session, Rome, May 27–29, 1982, IOCL, pp. 56–57.

36. De Merode quoted in Todd, "A History of the Use of Anabolic Steroids in Sport," 332.

37. See Hage, "Caffeine, Testosterone Banned for Olympians," 15, 17.

38. Voy and Deeter, *Drugs, Sport, and Politics*, 104.

39. Pound quoted in Randy Harvey, "IOC Official Questions Drug Testing in Track," *Los Angeles Times*, May 9, 1989. See also Voy and Deeter, *Drugs, Sport, and Politics*, 104.

40. See Voy and Deeter, *Drugs, Sport, and Politics*, 102–105.

41. These included one cyclist, one sprinter, one fencer, one shot-putter, and eleven

weightlifters. Their most prominent member was U.S. weightlifter Jeff Michaels. See Todd and Todd, "Significant Events in the History of Drug Testing and the Olympic Movement," 79.

42. See Frank Litsky, "Some U.S. Athletes Leave Games at Caracas amid Stiff Drug Tests," *New York Times,* August 24, 1983.

43. Emphasis in original. Dennis quoted in Craig Neff, "Caracas: A Scandal and a Warning," *Sports Illustrated,* September 5, 1983, 20.

44. Kelly comments in Proceedings of the Meetings of the USOC Administrative Committee and Executive Board, July 15–16, 1983, New York, USOCLA, p. 190.

45. See "Some on U.S. Squad at Caracas Failed Drug Tests before Games," *New York Times,* August 27, 1983.

46. Voy and Deeter, *Drugs, Sport, and Politics,* 102–103.

47. Ronald Reagan, "Remarks at the Annual Convention of the National Association of Evangelicals in Orlando, Florida," March 8, 1983. Downloaded from John T. Woolley and Gerhard Peters, *The American Presidency Project* [online]. Santa Barbara, CA, http://www.presidency.ucsb.edu/ws/?pid=41023.

48. Ronald Reagan, "Remarks at a Luncheon Meeting of the United States Olympic Committee in Los Angeles, California," March 3, 1983. Downloaded from John T. Woolley and Gerhard Peters, *The American Presidency Project* [online]. Santa Barbara, CA, http://www.presidency.ucsb.edu/ws/?pid=40995.

49. Bjarne Rostaing and Robert Sullivan, "Triumphs Tainted with Blood," *Sports Illustrated,* January 21, 1985, 14.

CHAPTER 6

1. See "The Daily Dope Dialogue," *Track and Field News,* February 1985, 52; Todd and Todd, "Significant Events in the History of Drug Testing and the Olympic Movement," 83–84.

2. Voy and Deeter, *Drugs, Sport, and Politics,* 89–90.

3. See "86 Athletes Tested Positive," *New York Times,* January 11, 1985. See also Todd, "A History of the Use of Anabolic Steroids in Sport," 334; "U.S. Olympic Group to Weight Drug Test Plan: 86 American Athletes Failed 1984 Screening," *Chronicle of Higher Education,* January 23, 1985. Prior to the 1984 Games, the public was told that all members of the U.S. track-and-field team had passed their drug tests at the Olympic trials. See "U.S. Track Olympians Pass Drug Tests," *New York Times,* July 18, 1984.

4. An award-winning study of the IOC's ascent as an economic power is provided in Robert Knight Barney, Stephen R. Wenn, and Scott G. Martyn, *Selling the Five Rings: The International Olympic Committee and the Rise of Olympic Commercialism,* rev. ed. (Salt Lake City: University of Utah Press, 2004).

5. The best biography of Samaranch is Miller, *Olympic Revolution.* See also Juan Antonio Samaranch and Robert Parienté, *The Samaranch Years: 1980–1994, Towards Olympic Unity* (Lausanne: International Olympic Committee, 1995).

6. These aspects of Samaranch's leadership are described in Peter Ueberroth, with Richard Levin and Amy Quinn, *Made in America: His Own Story* (New York: Fawcett Crest, 1987), 202.

7. Michael Payne, *Olympic Turnaround: How the Olympic Games Stepped Back*

from the Brink of Extinction to Become the World's Best Known Brand (Westport, CT: Praeger, 2006), 7.

8. Pound and Samaranch quoted from Pound, *Inside the Olympics,* 67.

9. On Ueberroth's leadership in Los Angeles, see Kenneth Reich, *Making It Happen: Peter Ueberroth and the 1984 Olympics* (Santa Barbara, CA: Capra Press, 1986). For the financial aspects of the Los Angeles Games, see in particular pages 87–104.

10. Ueberroth, *Made in America,* 334.

11. Usher's operational role in Los Angeles is discussed in Reich, *Making It Happen,* 69–86.

12. Patano quoted in Reich, *Making It Happen,* 31.

13. See "Drug Testing at Issue," *New York Times,* April 29, 1983. An anonymous member of the Los Angeles organizing committee admitted that this decision was related to the cost of testing; see Elliott Almond, Julie Cart, and Randy Harvey, "The Olympic Dope Sheet Is Redefined," *Los Angeles Times,* November 13, 1983. A clipping of this article can be found in IOC Medical Commission Records, Folder "IOC, Commission Médicale: Dopage—Correspondence et articles de presse, 1965–1977," IOCL.

14. Daly to de Merode, June 8, 1983, IOC Medical Commission Records, Folder "IOC, Méd. Comm., Los Angeles '84 medical matters, 1985–1986–1994," IOCL.

15. Ueberroth to Samaranch, November 14, 1983, IOC Medical Commission Records, Folder "Médicale: Dopage—Correspondence et articles de presse, 1965–1977," IOCL.

16. Ueberroth quoted in Jennings, *The New Lords of the Rings,* 238.

17. Drs. Hans Howald and Donike provided this scientific testimony, according to "Report on the Seminar of the Medical Commission of the IOC," September 25–October 2, 1983, IOC Medical Commission Records, Folder "IOC, SD1: Comm. Méd.: Rapp. Sessions, CE 1968–1984," IOCL. The final decision to test for caffeine and testosterone in Los Angeles is recorded in "Report of the IOC Medical Commission," November 24–25, 1983, IOC Medical Commission Records, Folder "IOC, SD1: Comm. Méd.: Rapp. Sessions, CE 1968–1984," IOCL. See also Annex 22, "Report of the Medical Commission Presented by Prince Alexandre De Merode, Chairman," in Minutes of the IOC General Session, Sarajevo, February 5–6, 1984, IOCL, pp. 90–91.

18. See Almond, Cart, and Harvey, "The Olympic Dope Sheet Is Redefined." For an early analysis of the future effect of hGH on sport, see Terry Todd, "Sports RX: The Use of Human Growth Hormone Poses a Grave Dilemma for Sport," *Sports Illustrated,* October 15, 1984, 8.

19. "Report of the IOC Medical Commission," November 24–25, 1983, IOC Medical Commission Records, Folder "IOC, SD1: Comm. Méd.: Rapp. Sessions, CE 1968–1984," IOCL.

20. Soviet officials cited unfair treatment in Los Angeles as one of the reasons for the Soviet boycott of the 1984 summer Olympics. See "Statement of the Soviet National Olympic Committee," May 8, 1984, reprinted in Edward H. Judge and John W. Langdon, eds., *The Cold War: A History through Documents* (Upper Saddle River, NJ: Prentice Hall, 1999), 220–221.

21. Ewald to de Merode, November 9, 1983, IOC Medical Commission Records, Folder "Los Angeles '84 Medical Matters, 1978–1983," IOCL.

22. Ueberroth quoted in Reich, *Making It Happen,* 222.

23. Lewis quoted in Lewis H. Carlson and John J. Fogarty, *Tales of Gold: An Oral*

History of the Summer Olympic Games Told by America's Gold Medal Winners (Chicago: Contemporary Books, 1987), 492.

24. Carraro and de Merode statements from Minutes of the IOC General Session, Los Angeles, July 25–26, 1984, IOCL, p. 23.

25. "Report of the Medical Commission Presented by Alexandre de Merode, Chairman," Minutes of the IOC General Session, Los Angeles, July 25–26, 1984, Annex 19, IOCL, p. 74.

26. Minutes of the IOC General Session, Los Angeles, July 25–26, 1984, IOCL, p. 23.

27. The medal totals for the Los Angeles Games are provided on the IOC internet website, www.olympic.org.

28. See Pound, *Inside the Olympics*, 67–68.

29. John Hoberman identifies IOC president Samaranch and medical commission head de Merode as the central figures of the cover-up. John M. Hoberman, "How Drug Testing Fails: The Politics of Doping Control," in *Significant Events in the History of Drug Testing and the Olympic Movement: 1960–1999,* ed. Wayne Wilson and Edward Derse (Champaign, IL: Human Kinetics, 2001), 244.

30. The best account of the destruction of the doping documents in Los Angeles is provided in Jim Ferstle, "Evolution and Politics of Drug Testing," in *Anabolic Steroids in Sport and Exercise,* ed. Charles E. Yesalis, 2nd ed. (Champaign, IL: Human Kinetics, 2000), 386–387.

31. Pound, *Inside the Olympics,* 68.

32. Kammerer quoted in Hoberman, "How Drug Testing Fails," 244.

33. Pound's description of himself quoted from Frank Deford, Kostya Kennedy, and Richard Deitsch, "Just Say No," *Sports Illustrated,* December 16, 2002, 48.

34. Pound, *Inside the Olympics,* 67.

35. Beckett quoted in Hoberman, "How Drug Testing Fails," 244.

36. This stance extended to future scholarship on the issue. Dr. Catlin wished to copublish his recollections of the episode (with Craig Kammerer, the assistant director of the laboratory at the Los Angeles Games) in a medical journal, but was prohibited by de Merode. Catlin asserted, "I would not still be a member of the IOC medical commission if I had published a report without the co-operation of the prince." Catlin quoted in Jennings, *The New Lords of the Rings,* 242. This work includes a useful discussion of the cover-up (pp. 237–243).

37. See Robert McG. Thomas Jr., "U.S.O.C. Checking Use of Transfusions," *New York Times,* January 10, 1985.

38. This description of "blood doping" can be found in Houlihan, *Dying to Win,* 87–88.

39. Thomas, "U.S.O.C. Checking Use of Transfusions." For a contemporaneous legal analysis concerning the possible prohibition of blood doping, see G. Legwold, "Blood Doping and the Letter of the Law," *Physician and Sportsmedicine* 13 (March 1985): 37–38.

40. "Cycle Group Bans Use of Blood Doping," *New York Times,* January 19, 1985. This article also describes the sanctions handed out to the officials involved in the scandal: Eddy Borysewicz, a team coach, and Ed Burke, director of the federation's Elite Athlete Program, were both suspended without pay for thirty days and received letters

of reprimand. Former USCF president Mike Fraysse was also demoted from first vice president to third vice president of the organization.

41. Minutes of the Meeting of the Administrative Committee of the United States Olympic Committee, May 4, 1985, Chicago, USOCLA, p. 140.

42. Harvey G. Klein, "Blood Transfusions and Athletics: Games People Play," *New England Journal of Medicine* 312, no. 13 (March 1985): 854–856. See also Richard D. Lyons, "Expert Urges Ban on Blood Doping," *New York Times,* March 28, 1985. In January 1985, the Food and Drug Administration also requested that the Justice Department begin an investigation of the illegal "black market" distribution of anabolic steroids. See Todd, "A History of the Use of Anabolic Steroids in Sport," 338.

43. Carlgren's argument over the importance of doping to the direction of the Olympic movement is provided in Minutes of the IOC General Session, December 1–2, 1984, Lausanne, IOCL, p. 13.

44. "Report of the IOC Medical Commission to the 90th Session of the IOC," appended as Annex 11 to Minutes of the IOC General Session, June 4–6, 1985, Berlin, IOCL, p. 85. In addition, on page 22 of the minutes of this meeting, Dr. Eduardo Hay supported de Merode's position, even though "it was not possible for the time being to provide that blood doping had been practiced" in Los Angeles.

45. Minutes of the IOC General Session, June 4–6, 1985, Berlin, IOCL, p. 21.

46. See "Drugs Used," *New York Times,* August 6, 1984.

47. See de Merode circular to International Sports Federations, National Olympic Committees, and IOC Accredited Dope Control Laboratories, May 31, 1985, attached to Annex 11, Minutes of the IOC General Session, June 4–6, 1985, Berlin, IOCL, p. 21.

48. A description of beta-blockers is provided in Houlihan, *Dying to Win,* 91–92.

49. Minutes of the IOC General Session, June 4–6, 1985, Berlin, IOCL, p. 21. See also de Merode circular to International Sports Federations, National Olympic Committees, and IOC Accredited Dope Control Laboratories, May 31, 1985.

50. Clark and Prouty quoted in Michael Goodwin, "U.S.O.C. to Seek More Tests for Drugs," *New York Times,* March 24, 1985.

51. Even then, only twenty of the thirty-eight national governing bodies supported the plan. See "U.S.O.C. to Begin Tests," *New York Times,* June 25, 1985.

52. Ibid.

53. See Voy and Deeter, *Drugs, Sport, and Politics,* 111–112.

54. Vera Rich, "Mortality of Soviet Athletes," *Nature* 311 (October 4, 1984): 402–403. See also Hoberman, *Mortal Engines,* 3; "Early Deaths of Soviet Athletes Due to Steroids? Magazine Cites 59 Cases in Which Banned Drugs Proved Fatal at Young Age," *Los Angeles Times,* September 6, 1984.

55. See Voy and Deeter, *Drugs, Sport, and Politics,* 106–108.

56. The replacements were Dr. Birginia Mikhaylova and Dr. Arne Ljungqvist. See Voy and Deeter, *Drugs, Sport, and Politics,* 108.

57. See Vyv Simson and Andrew Jennings, *Dishonored Games: Corruption, Money and Greed at the Olympics* (New York: S.P.I. Books, 1992), 169.

58. Samaranch quoted in "Executive Board Meeting of December," *Olympic Review,* January 1988, 21.

59. "Speech by H. E. Juan Antonio Samaranch, President of the IOC (93rd Session)," *Olympic Review,* March 1988, 82, 83.

60. See Michael Janofsky, "I.O.C. Criticizes Federation Steroids Rule," *New York Times,* September 8, 1989.

61. Francis and Lyon quoted in Charlie Francis with Jeff Coplon, *Speed Trap: Inside the Biggest Scandal in Olympic History* (New York: St. Martin's Press, 1990), 1.

62. Pound, *Inside the Olympics,* 49. Pound's recollections of the 1988 Games are also recounted in Richard W. Pound, *Five Rings over Korea: The Secret Negotiations behind the 1988 Olympic Games in Seoul* (Boston: Little, Brown, 1994), but he makes little reference to drugs.

63. Moses quoted in "Johnson Home in Disgrace: Canada Bans Him for Life. Can't Run for Country or Get Funds," *Los Angeles Times,* September 27, 1988.

64. Heidebrecht quoted in "The Seoul Games, Day 12 Notes: Johnson Advertisements Canceled," *Los Angeles Times,* September 28, 1988.

65. Ibid.

66. See Francis, *Speed Trap,* 7.

67. Worrall quoted in Michael Janofsky, "Johnson Loses Gold to Lewis after Drug Test," *New York Times,* September 27, 1988.

68. See Alfred E. Senn, *Power, Politics, and the Olympic Games* (Champaign, IL: Human Kinetics, 1999), 229.

69. The ship was the *Michail Shalokhov.* See Voy and Deeter, *Drugs, Sport, and Politics,* 89.

70. "Team Lifted after 2d Drug Test Is Failed," *New York Times,* September 24, 1988; "Weight Lifter Used Drug," *New York Times,* September 29, 1988.

71. Voy and Deeter, *Drugs, Sport, and Politics,* 109–110, 112.

72. President Samaranch asserted at a summer 1989 IOC general session, for example, that "in Seoul, the Medical Commission had proved how seriously it took its work; the Olympic Movement was thus showing an example to [other] sports organizations." Minutes of the IOC General Session, August 30–September 1, 1989, [San Juan?], Puerto Rico, p. 12, copy on file at the Todd-McLean Physical Culture Collection, H. J. Lutcher Stark Center for Physical Culture and Sport, University of Texas at Austin. I thank Jan and Terry Todd for allowing me access to their collection.

73. Pound and Samaranch quoted in Janofsky, "Johnson Loses Gold to Lewis after Drug Test." See also Todd and Todd, "Significant Events in the History of Drug Testing and the Olympic Movement," 90.

74. Voy quoted in Michael Janofsky and Peter Alfano, "Drug Use by Athletes Runs Free Despite Tests," *New York Times,* November 17, 1988.

75. "Canadian Inquiry," *New York Times,* October 6, 1988.

76. A brief description of these events is provided in Varda Burstyn, *The Rites of Men: Manhood, Politics, and the Culture of Sport* (Toronto: University of Toronto Press, 1999), 221.

77. Charles Dubin, *Commission of Inquiry into the Use of Drugs and Banned Practices Intended to Increase Athletic Performance* (Ottawa: Canadian Government Publishing Centre, 1990), xx.

78. Ibid., 518.

79. Worrall quoted in Janofsky, "Johnson Loses Gold to Lewis after Drug Test."

80. Dubin, *Commission of Inquiry,* 519.

81. Pound and Worrall quoted in Janofsky, "Johnson Loses Gold to Lewis after Drug Test."

82. "Towards an Anti-Doping Charter," *Olympic Review,* August 1988, 350. A draft of the charter is provided in "International Olympic Charter against Doping in Sport," *Olympic Review,* November 1988, 628–631.

83. "Report from the Commissions," *Olympic Review,* November 1988, 618.

84. "Speech by H. E. Juan Antonio Samaranch, President of the International Olympic Committee, Moscow, 21st November 1988," *Olympic Review,* December 1988, 670.

85. See Robert Edelman, *Serious Fun: A History of Spectator Sports in the U.S.S.R.* (New York: Oxford University Press, 1993), 222–223.

86. According to a scholar of Bulgarian sport, "Bulgaria made a serious attempt [in the 1980s] to rebuild, at least morally, its national identity, in sharp contrast to Brezhnev's doctrine for limited national sovereignty." Vassil Girginov, "Bulgarian Sport Policy, 1945–1989: A Strategic Relations Approach," *International Journal of the History of Sport* 26, no. 4 (March 2009): 530.

87. Ter-Ovanesyan quoted in Jim Riordan, "Playing to New Rules: Soviet Sport and Perestroika," *Soviet Studies* 42, no. 1 (January 1990): 137.

88. Coupat quoted in Michael Janofsky, "Drug Plan Gains Approval," *New York Times,* November 25, 1988.

89. Ibid. The details of the agreement are provided in María Tai Wolff, "Playing by the Rules? A Legal Analysis of the United States Olympic Committee–Soviet Olympic Committee Doping Control Agreement," *Stanford Journal of International Law* 25, no. 2 (Spring 1989): 611–646.

90. See "11 Nations in Drug Test Accord," *New York Times,* December 14, 1989.

91. Excerpts of address by Mikhail Gorbachev, 43rd U.N. General Assembly Session, December 7, 1988, available from the Cold War Files of the Cold War International History Project, http://www.wilsoncenter.org/coldwarfiles/index.cfm?fuse action=home.flash).

92. "Commission Reports," *Olympic Review,* September–October 1989, 443. The official minutes of the IOC general session only briefly mention the new doping subcommittee. See Minutes of the IOC General Session, August 30–September 1, 1989, [San Juan?], Puerto Rico, p. 11, copy on file at the Todd-McLean Physical Culture Collection, H. J. Lutcher Stark Center for Physical Culture and Sport, University of Texas at Austin.

93. After the 1988 Seoul Olympics, de Merode remarked on the tenuousness of the medical commission's links with the international federations. He said that "the Medical Commission did have contacts with the IFs, but that these were not always simple." Minutes of the IOC General Session, August 30–September 1, 1989, [San Juan?], Puerto Rico, p. 12, copy on file at the Todd-McLean Physical Culture Collection, H. J. Lutcher Stark Center for Physical Culture and Sport, University of Texas at Austin.

94. Richard W. Pound, "Reflections on Cheating in Sport," *Olympic Review,* August 1989, 390.

CHAPTER 7

1. For an early review of changes in the GDR sport system, consult John M. Hoberman, "The Transformation of East German Sport," *Journal of Sport History* 17, no. 1 (Spring 1990): 62–68.

2. In a 1992 book, Olympic specialist John A. Lucas predicted several alternatives for how Olympic doping policy might evolve in the 1990s. See John A. Lucas, *Future of the Olympic Games* (Champaign, IL: Human Kinetics, 1992), 110–111.

3. The existing scholarship on the establishment and early history of the World Anti-Doping Agency utilizes few primary sources of evidence. For an examination of this subject based almost entirely on secondary works, see Hanstad, Smith, and Waddington, "The Establishment of the World Anti-Doping Agency," 227–249. See also Ulrik Wagner, "The World Anti-Doping Agency: Constructing a Hybrid Organisation in Permanent Stress (Dis)order?" *International Journal of Sport Policy* 1 (July 2009): 183–201; Barrie Houlihan, "Harmonising Anti-Doping Policy: The Role of the World Anti-Doping Agency," in *Doping and Public Policy,* edited by John M. Hoberman and Verner Møller (Odense: University Press of Southern Denmark, 2004), 19–30. A broader study of the growth of an international approach to doping regulation is provided by Houlihan in "Anti-Doping Policy in Sport: The Politics of International Policy Coordination," *Public Administration* 77, no. 2 (Summer 1999): 311–334.

4. Pound quoted in Houlihan, "Anti-Doping Policy in Sport," 106.

5. De Merode quoted in Miller, *Olympic Revolution,* 151.

6. Samaranch quoted in Hoberman, "How Drug Testing Fails," 266.

7. Juan Antonio Samaranch, "Maintaining Our Impetus," *Olympic Review,* January 1990, 5.

8. De Merode suggested the possibility of "a flying medical analysis laboratory" at a 1989 IOC general session. The medical commission chair elaborated that "the mobile laboratory would be a complementary laboratory and would be used where no laboratory existed. This system would be of use to the IFs since they could thus avoid unnecessary investments. It would be used for out-of-competition controls." See Minutes of the IOC General Session, [San Juan?], Puerto Rico, August 30 and September 1, 1989, p. 11, copy on file at the Todd-McLean Physical Culture Collection, H. J. Lutcher Stark Center for Physical Culture and Sport, University of Texas at Austin.

9. De Merode quoted in "Flying Laboratory Operational Soon," *Olympic Review,* January 1990, 6.

10. Armstrong quoted in Ferstle, "Evolution and Politics of Drug Testing," 393.

11. Juan Antonio Samaranch, "Speech by H. E. Mr Juan Antonio Samaranch, IOC President," *Olympic Review,* May–June 1990, 243.

12. The early history of the court is addressed in Richard McLaren, "A New Order: Athletes Rights and the Court of Arbitration at the Olympic Games," *Olympika: The International Journal of Olympic Studies* 7 (1998): 1–24; and Matthieu Reeb, "The Court of Arbitration for Sport (CAS)," in *Digest of CAS Awards, 1986–1998,* ed. Matthieu Reeb (Berne: Staempfli SA, 1998), xxiii–xxxi. For a brief overview of the organizational structure and procedural mechanisms of the CAS, consult Antonio Buti and Saul Fridman, *Drugs, Sport and the Law* (Mudgeeraba, Australia: Scribblers Publishing, 2001), 97–100. A larger overview is provided in Ian S. Blackshaw, Robert C. R. Siekmann, and Janwillem Soek, eds., *The Court of Arbitration for Sport, 1984–2004* (The Hague: TMC Asser Press, 2006). See also Jean-Loup Chappelet and Brenda Kübler-Mabbott, *The International Olympic Committee and the Olympic System: The Governance of World Sport* (New York: Routledge, 2008), 128–132.

13. Anita L. DeFrantz, "Which Rules? International Sport and Doping in the 21st Century," *Houston Journal of International Law* 31, no. 1 (Fall 2008): 20.

14. Ibid., 21.

15. Emphasis added. Court of Arbitration for Sport, Advisory Opinion No. 86/02 (CAS 1986), cited in Frank Oschütz, "Harmonization of Anti-Doping Code through Arbitration: The Case Law of the Court of Arbitration for Sport," *Marquette Sports Law Review* 12 (Spring 2002): 680–681.

16. A rationale for the CAS was best stated by one of its arbitrators in Tricia Kavanagh, "The Doping Cases and the Need for the International Court of Arbitration for Sport (CAS)," *University of New South Wales Law Journal* 22 (Summer 1999): 721–745. On athletes' rights, see Barrie Houlihan, "Civil Rights, Doping Control and the World Anti-Doping Code," *Sport in Society* 7, no. 3 (Autumn 2004): 420–437.

17. Michael Janofsky, "Barnes Claims Testing for Steroids Was Flawed," *New York Times,* November 7, 1990.

18. Mark Asher and Christine Brennan, "TAC Clears Reynolds of Steroid Use Charge: International Hearing His Next Hurdle," *Washington Post,* October 5, 1991.

19. See Ferstle, "Evolution and Politics of Drug Testing," 396.

20. LaShutka quoted in Asher and Brennan, "TAC Clears Reynolds of Steroid Use Charge."

21. Reynolds quoted in Asher and Brennan, "TAC Clears Reynolds of Steroid Use Charge."

22. In terms of TAC's reputation, Edwin Moses, chair of the USOC Substance Abuse Committee, alleged that officials affiliated with the body deliberately provided insufficient information at doping hearings held in 1989 in order to clear six American athletes of drug charges. See Voy and Deeter, *Drugs, Sport, and Politics,* 106.

23. Christie quoted in "Christie Slams US Decision on Reynolds," *Herald Sun* (Melbourne), June 18, 1991. See Hoberman, *Testosterone Dreams,* 226.

24. Reynolds first won an injunction requiring the IAAF to rescind his suspension in *Reynolds v. International Amateur Athletic Federation,* 841 F. Supp. 1444 (S.D. Ohio 1992). A stay on the injunction was subsequently ordered by the U.S. Sixth Circuit Court of Appeals in *Reynolds v. International Amateur Athletic Federation,* 1992 U.S. App. LEXIS 14058 (U.S. 6th Cir. 1992). The Sixth Circuit was itself reversed by the United States Supreme Court in *Reynolds v. International Amateur Athletic Federation,* 505 U.S. 1301 (U.S. Supreme Court 1992). See also Glenn M. Wong, *Essentials of Sports Law,* 3rd ed. (Westport, CT: Praeger, 2002), 305.

25. For the award, see Wong, *Essentials of Sports Law,* 305.

26. De Merode quoted in "IOC to Review Procedures to Stem Drug Test Suits," *Washington Post,* December 8, 1992.

27. Ibid.

28. The award was reversed in *Reynolds v. International Amateur Athletic Federation,* 23 F.3d 1110 (6th Cir. 1994).

29. De Merode quoted in "IOC to Review Procedures to Stem Drug Test Suits."

30. The athletes included six-time Olympic gold medalist swimmer Kristin Otto; 1988 silver and gold medalist swimmer Heike Friedrich; 1988 Olympic shot-put champion Ulf Timmermann; 1988 Olympic discus champion Juergen Schult; 1988 gold medal decathlete Christian Schenck; silver medalist Torsten Voss; 1988 silver and bronze medalist jumper Heike Dreschler; and Dagmar Hase, who would go on to win seven Olympic medals in the 1990s. Michael Janofsky, "Drug Use by Prominent Ath-

letes Reported," *New York Times,* November 29, 1990. See also Todd and Todd, "Significant Events in the History of Drug Testing and the Olympic Movement," 97.

31. Franke and Berendonk, "Hormonal Doping and Androgenization of Athletes," 1263.

32. Berendonk, *Doping Dokumente.*

33. De Merode quoted in Hoberman, "How Drug Testing Fails," 244.

34. See "Germanys Closer to Olympic Merger," *Washington Post,* August 13, 1990; "Olympics: Backing for Germans," *New York Times,* August 17, 1990; Marc Fischer, "IOC Supports Idea of Berlin Games," *Washington Post,* January 23, 1990.

35. Samaranch quoted in Peter Herrmann, "Germany's 'Miracle Machine' Is Left in the Blocks," *New York Times,* November 4, 1990.

36. Samaranch quoted in Hoberman, *Testosterone Dreams,* 247. See also Hoberman, *Mortal Engines,* 267.

37. Samaranch quoted in Miller, *Olympic Revolution,* 150.

38. Juan Antonio Samaranch, "The IOC President's Speech at the Opening of the 97th Session," *Olympic Review,* July 1991, 309–310.

39. "Important Medical Meetings This Autumn," *Olympic Review,* September 1991, 433.

40. Radford quoted in "Athletes Want Drug Bans," *Courier-Mail* (Brisbane), September 26, 1991.

41. Dupre quoted in Norman Da Costa, "Illegal Drug Use by Athletes Reported on Rise in Canada," *Toronto Star,* September 25, 1991. In a similar argument, Sergio Fantini, then president of Chile's national Olympic committee, wrote in February 1990, "Doping can destroy athletes and therefore the movement. Massive education first, and along with it strict enforcement [are] the only way out of this nightmare." Quoted in Lucas, *Future of the Olympic Games,* 105.

42. "The Executive Board and the Summer IFs in Barcelona," *Olympic Review,* May 1991, 187.

43. See Allan R. Gold, "Albertville '92: I.O.C. Looks at Use of Blood Tests," *New York Times,* February 7, 1992. An alternative to erythropoietin introduces an athlete's own recycled blood cells (or those of another) into the body in order to boost the amount of oxygen in the competitor's body. Both techniques are discussed in Houlihan, *Dying to Win,* 87–88.

44. "Commission Reports," *Olympic Review,* July 1991, 322.

45. De Merode quoted in "The Executive Board in Berlin," *Olympic Review,* October–November 1991, 489.

46. Catlin quoted in Michael Janofsky, "Olympics: Sophisticated Doping Begets More Testing," *New York Times,* July 19, 1992.

47. Nurikian quoted in Vassil Girginov, "Creating a Corporate Anti-Doping Culture: The Role of Bulgarian Sports Governing Bodies," *Sport in Society* 9, no. 2 (April 2006): 260.

48. The other two athletes were Grit Breuer, a 1991 World Track-and-Field Championships silver medalist, and former 100-meter and 200-meter world champion Silke Moller. See Todd and Todd, "Significant Events in the History of Drug Testing and the Olympic Movement," 98–99; William Oscar Johnson and Anita Verschoth, "Testy Times in Germany," *Sports Illustrated,* March 9, 1992, 51–52.

49. Springstein and Grau quoted in Marc Fischer, "Germany Has Everything—

Except for Harmony," *Washington Post,* July 22, 1992. John Hoberman perceives little substance to the allegations made by former GDR sports officials and athletes of discrimination in the newly unified country. In contrast, he argues that shared values regarding performance enhancement by the GDR and West Germany led to a quick and easy integration of the two sports establishments. See John M. Hoberman, "The Reunification of German Sports Medicine, 1989–2002," *Quest* 45, no. 2 (May 1993): 277–285.

50. Johnson and Verschoth, "Testy Times in Germany," 51–52.

51. Vrijman quoted in Johnson and Verschoth, "Testy Times in Germany," 51–52.

52. Ramsay quoted in "Track and Field: African Official Seeks Help on Drug Detection," *New York Times,* September 7, 1993.

53. Jacomini quoted in Dick Patrick and Gary Mihoces, "Krabbe Cleared to Run by German Federation," *USA Today,* March 31, 1993.

54. See Mark Hayes and Michael Hiestand, "Krabbe Case," *USA Today,* August 24, 1993, international edition.

55. See Furthermore, *Washington Post,* May 18, 1995. After initially appealing the decision by the regional court, the IAAF later dropped its appeal. See "Track and Field: I.A.A.F. Drops Appeal on Krabbe," *New York Times,* January 29, 1997.

56. Thompson quoted in "Swimmers' Drug Tests in Spotlight," *Washington Post,* July 28, 1992.

57. Andrew Davies and Andrew Saxton were the two British weightlifters who tested positive for Clenbuterol. See Beth Tuschak, "British Want IOC Heads to Clarify Doping Rules," *USA Today,* November 6, 1992. A third British athlete, Jason Livingston, the 60-meter European indoor champion, was also suspended after failing a precompetition test for anabolic steroids. See "3 U.K. Athletes Sent Home in Doping Scandal," *Toronto Star,* July 30, 1992.

58. Minutes of UNESCO General Conference, August 1991, Paris, Item 6.7 of Provisional Agenda, p. 2, http://unesdoc.unesco.org/ulis/index.shtml. A passage of this document declared: "The only instrument of international scope—the Charter of the International Olympic Committee—despite its wide-scale geographical coverage, does not have the authority of a document emanating from an intergovernmental organization."

59. UNESCO, "Study on the Technical and Legal Aspects of the Desirability of Drawing Up an International Instrument to Combat Doping in Sport, Submitted to First Meeting of the Group of Experts," Paipa, Colombia, December 7, 1992, p. 7, http://unesdoc.unesco.org/ulis/index.shtml.

60. Carrard and de Merode quoted in "Olympic Sports Set to Unify Doping Rules, Penalties," *Washington Post,* June 22, 1993.

61. DeFrantz, "Which Rules?" 22.

CHAPTER 8

1. Jinxia Dong, *Women, Sport, and Society in Modern China: Holding Up More than Half the Sky* (Portland, OR: Frank Cass, 2003), 142–143.

2. Xiong quoted in Filip Bondy, "Barcelona: Swimming. Too Good? Too Fast? Drug Rumors Stalk Chinese," *New York Times,* July 31, 1992.

3. Chalmers and Clement quoted in Randy Starkman, "Chinese Track Success Sparks Doping Questions," *Toronto Star,* August 17, 1993.

4. For the reaction to the events in Stuttgart, consult Darcy C. Plymire, "Too Much, Too Fast, Too Soon: Chinese Women Runners, Accusations of Steroid Use, and the Politics of American Track and Field," *Sociology of Sport Journal* 16, no. 2 (June 1999): 155–173.

5. Chalmers and Pells quoted in Randy Starkman, "Athletes Call for Doping Crackdown on Chinese Runners," *Toronto Star,* August 23, 1993.

6. The International Swimming Federation (FINA) was not given information on the tests by Chinese authorities. FINA officials became aware of the information during a 1995 visit to the PRC. See David Galluzzi, "The Doping Crisis in International Athletic Competition: Lessons from the Chinese Doping Scandal in Women's Swimming," *Seton Hall Journal of Sport Law* 10 (Winter 2000): 77–78.

7. De Merode quoted in Hoberman, "How Drug Testing Fails," 244. Eleven Chinese competitors failed drug tests at the competition. See "China to Investigate Doping," *New York Times,* December 1, 1994.

8. Carrard quoted in Jennings, *The New Lords of the Rings,* 234.

9. See Kidd, Edelman, and Brownell, "Comparative Analysis of Doping Scandals," 174. The notion of racist interpretations of Chinese success was also articulated during the 1994 Asian Games by the Olympic Council of Asia. The council blamed "racism and the western media for untrue doping slurs against Chinese athletes." Quoted in Jennings, *The New Lords of the Rings,* 232.

10. Quoted in Kidd, Edelman, and Brownell, "Comparative Analysis of Doping Scandals," 174.

11. Quoted in Galluzzi, "The Doping Crisis in International Athletic Competition," 80–81.

12. The investigation is addressed in "China to Investigate Doping." Beckman's quote comes from this article.

13. See Galluzzi, "The Doping Crisis in International Athletic Competition," 80.

14. See Furthermore, *Washington Post,* February 13, 1995.

15. Zaleski quoted in Karen Allen, "Group's Anti-Drug Action 'Thrills' U.S. Swimming," *USA Today,* February 14, 1995.

16. Kidd, Edelman, and Brownell, "Comparative Analysis of Doping Scandals," 176–177.

17. See Galluzzi, "The Doping Crisis in International Athletic Competition," 81.

18. Al Gore, "Al Gore: Promoting Preventive Education," *Olympic Review,* February–March 1995, 44.

19. Walker quoted in "USOC Passes Stiff Antidrug Program," *USA Today,* April 15, 1996.

20. Schultz quoted in Debbie Becker and Dick Patrick, "USOC Control of Testing Might Come after Atlanta," *USA Today,* October 6, 1995. These policies had been at least a year in the making. See also Christine Brennan, "USOC Eyes Tougher Tests: Wants No-Notice Drug Tests in All Sports," *Washington Post,* September 9, 1995; Athelia Knight, "USOC: Atlanta Too Soon for Stronger Drug Testing," *Washington Post,* October 6, 1995; and Mike Dodd, "USOC Ready to Approve No-Notice Drug Testing," *USA Today,* April 12, 1996.

21. Cantwell quoted in "Inside the Olympic Medical Tent," *Physician and Sports-*

medicine 24, no. 6 (June 1996): 28. For the numbers relating to this massive undertaking, see Thomas Heath, "Drug Testing Performance Enhanced: High-Tech Equipment, Better Methods, But Will Abusers Slip Through?" *Washington Post,* April 23, 1996.

22. Hale quoted in Ferstle, "Evolution and Politics of Drug Testing," 375.

23. See "The Olympian Battle over hGH," *Sports Illustrated,* October 30, 1995. In the end, the IOC did not use a test for human growth hormone until the 2004 Games in Athens. See M. Saugy et al., "Human Growth Hormone Doping in Sport," *British Journal of Sports Medicine* 40, no. 1, Supplement I (July, 2006): I37.

24. Cassell quoted in Mike Fish, "Atlanta Games: 111 Days. Drug Test," *Atlanta Journal and Constitution,* March 30, 1996.

25. See Ferstle, "Evolution and Politics of Drug Testing," 390.

26. DeFrantz, "Which Rules?" 23.

27. Hybl quoted in Robbi Pickeral and Rodney Page, "USOC Asks FBI to Investigate Web Site," *St. Petersburg Times,* December 9, 1997.

28. See "USOC Imposing Tougher Drug Tests," *St. Petersburg Times,* December 13, 1997.

29. See Karen Rosen, "Foschi Files Lawsuit in Steroid Case," *Atlanta Journal and Constitution,* February 6, 1996.

30. Zaleski quoted in Steve Berkowitz, "Muddied Waters Cloud Swimmer's Case: Neither Foschi nor U.S. Swimming Happy with Penalty for Positive Drug Test," *Washington Post,* February 11, 1996.

31. See Christine Brennan, "Suspension on Foschi Is Lifted: U.S. Officials Reverse Ban on Swimmer," *Washington Post,* February 24, 1996.

32. See Athelia Knight, "Arbitration Panel Rules for Foschi," *Washington Post,* April 9, 1996.

33. See "Swimming: Foschi Is Banned by International Group," *New York Times,* June 25, 1996.

34. See "Foschi Cleared to Compete," *New York Times,* June 19, 1997.

35. The CAS decision regarding bromantan was not published. The case was *Korneev & Gouliev v. International Olympic Committee* (Unreported, CAS Appeal Panel, August 4, 1996). It is referenced in note 90 of Kavanagh, "The Doping Cases and the Need for the International Court of Arbitration for Sport (CAS)," 742. See also Hoberman, "How Drug Testing Fails," 247. The Atlanta Games were the first to feature a mandatory arbitration agreement for competitors. On their entry forms, athletes signed a provision stating, "The decisions of the CAS [shall] be final, nonappealable and enforceable." Quoted in Mary K. FitzGerald, "The Court of Arbitration for Sport: Dealing with Doping and Due Process during the Olympics," *Sports Law Journal* 7 (Spring 2000): 238.

36. Rochat quoted in Andy Miller and M. A. J. McKenna, "Court Returns Medals, Changes Doping Scoreboard," *Atlanta Journal and Constitution,* August 5, 1996. See also "IOC Says It Will Ignore 5 Positive Steroid Tests," *Atlanta Journal and Constitution,* November 28, 1996.

37. Pound, *Inside the Olympics,* 68.

38. See Jere Longman, "Track and Field: I.A.A.F. Reduces Doping Bans," *New York Times,* August 1, 1997.

39. Carrard quoted in Furthermore, *Washington Post,* September 1, 1997.

40. Pound, *Inside the Olympics,* 69.

41. Ibid. Samaranch's comments are also discussed in Hoberman, "How Drug Testing Fails," 266.

42. Richard W. Pound and John M. Hoberman, "Olympic Roundtable," *Olympika: The International Journal of Olympic Studies* 10 (2001): 76.

43. De Merode quoted in Christopher P. Winner, "Sports Doping Crisis Faces a Crossroads," *USA Today*, September 28, 1998, international edition.

44. See Pound, *Inside the Olympics*, 69–70.

45. De Merode quoted in "IOC Anti-Drug Agency on the Drawing Board," *Chicago Sun-Times*, August 20, 1998.

46. See Irvin Molotsky, "Justice Department Begins Investigation of Salt Lake Bid," *New York Times*, December 24, 1998.

47. On the effect of these episodes, see Hoberman, *Testosterone Dreams*, 260–262. On the effect of the 1998 Tour de France scandal on IOC doping policy, see Hanstad, Smith, and Waddington, "The Establishment of the World Anti-Doping Agency," 227–249, and especially pp. 228–231. For an evaluation of the complex social system involved in the distribution and use of performance-enhancing substances during the 1998 Tour, consult Ivan Waddington, *Sport, Health, and Drugs: A Critical Sociological Perspective* (London: Taylor & Francis, 2000): 153–169. In April 1999, U.S. Congressman Henry Waxman introduced legislation aimed at forcing the IOC to reform its policies. See Remarks by Congressman Henry A. Waxman, The International Olympic Committee Reform Act, *Congressional Record (Extension of Remarks)*, 106th Congress, 1st sess., vol. 145, April 12, 1999 (Washington, DC: U.S. Government Printing Office, 1999), E 607. In terms of the rising public scrutiny of the IOC around this time, it is notable that IOC president Samaranch felt it necessary to testify before the U.S. Congress in December 1999 regarding the Salt Lake City bid scandal. See Robert Knight Barney, "Mr. Samaranch Goes to Washington: Protecting IOC Stakes in the American Corporate World," in *Bridging Three Centuries: Intellectual Crossroads and the Modern Olympic Movement. Fifth International Symposium for Olympic Research*, ed. Kevin B. Wamsley, Scott G. Martyn, Gordon H. MacDonald, and Robert Knight Barney (London, ON: International Centre for Olympic Studies, 2000), 29–36.

48. DeFrantz, "Which Rules?" 16.

49. Juan Antonio Samaranch, "The Fight against Doping," *Olympic Review*, October–November 1998, 3.

50. Vereen quoted in Dick Patrick, "IOC Drug Chief's Proposal Blasted," *USA Today*, February 1, 1999.

51. See "The World Conference on Doping in Sport," *Olympic Review*, October–November 1998, 9.

52. "Lausanne Declaration," *Olympic Review*, February–March 1999, 17–18.

53. An excellent analysis of the IOC's early conception of the proposed anti-doping authority is provided in John M. Hoberman, "Offering the Illusion of Reform on Drugs," *New York Times*, January 10, 1999. See also Kate Noble, Robert Kroon, and Tandy Nigel, "No Medals for the IOC," *Time South Pacific*, February 15, 1999, 62.

54. Banks quoted in Waddington, *Sport, Health, and Drugs*, 191.

55. McCaffrey quoted in Richard Sandomir, "I.O.C.'s Drug Plan Criticized at Hearing," *New York Times*, October 21, 1999. See also Todd and Todd, "Significant Events in the History of Drug Testing and the Olympic Movement," 108–109.

56. Pound, *Inside the Olympics,* 72–73.

57. Ibid., 73.

58. On Banks's original preference, see Waddington, *Sport, Health, and Drugs,* 191.

59. A brief history of WADA is provided on the organization's internet website, http://www.wada-ama.org/en/index.ch2.

60. "World Anti-Doping Agency," *Olympic Review,* February–March 2000, 5–6.

61. Minutes of the Inaugural Meeting of the Foundation Board of the World Anti-Doping Agency (WADA), January 13, 2000, p. 1, http://www.wada-ama.org/en/index .ch2.

62. A 2004 assessment of WADA addresses the challenges that it faced during the first decade of the twenty-first century. See Houlihan, "Harmonising Anti-Doping Policy," 19–30. The position that genetic modification is a natural—and perhaps even welcome—step in elite sport is best argued in Miah, *Genetically Modified Athletes.* A brief elucidation of the future of doping in elite sport is also provided in Hoberman, *Testosterone Dreams,* 274–275.

CHAPTER 9

1. Samaranch quoted in "Samaranch: Doping Is a Fact," *New York Times,* July 2, 2001.

2. The television contracts for the 2000 Sydney Games are outlined in Barney, Wenn, and Martyn, *Selling the Five Rings,* 4–5.

3. Pound, *Inside Dope,* 179.

4. National Center on Addiction and Substance Abuse at Columbia University, *Winning at Any Cost: Doping in Olympic Sports* (New York: 2000), 13.

5. Ibid., ii.

6. Ibid., 3.

7. Coderre quoted in James Christie, "'Do It Right' Anti-Drug Watchdog Warned: Future of Olympics on Line, Coderre Says," *Globe and Mail* (Toronto), January 13, 2000.

8. Minutes of the Inaugural Meeting of the Foundation Board of the World Anti-Doping Agency (WADA), January 13, 2000, Lausanne, p. 1, http://www.wada-ama .org/en/.

9. Pound and Hoberman, "Olympic Roundtable," 75–76, 78. Churchill's speech was made on October 29, 1941, to the students at Harrow School.

10. Dick Pound recalls Samaranch's explanation in Pound, *Inside the Olympics,* 74.

11. Pound played a key role in negotiating the set of contracts with the National Broadcasting Company for the rights to broadcast the 2004, 2006, and 2008 Olympics. See Stephen R. Wenn, "Riding into the Sunset: Richard Pound, Dick Ebersol, and Long-Term Olympic Television Contracts," in *Bridging Three Centuries: Intellectual Crossroads and the Modern Olympic Movement. Fifth International Symposium for Olympic Research,* ed. Kevin B. Wamsley, Scott G. Martyn, Gordon H. MacDonald, and Robert Knight Barney (London, ON: International Centre for Olympic Studies, September 2000), 37–50. For Pound's role in the Salt Lake City bid scandal, con-

sult Stephen R. Wenn and Scott G. Martyn, "'Tough Love': Richard Pound, David D'Alessandro, and the Salt Lake City Olympics Bid Scandal," *Sport in History* 26, no. 1 (April 2006): 69–90.

12. Pound, *Inside the Olympics*, x–xi.

13. Pound, *Inside Dope*, 2.

14. Pound quoted in Michael McCarthy, "Profile: Richard W. Pound, QC-Chairman of WADA," *Lancet* 366 (December 2005): S20.

15. Minutes of the Inaugural Meeting of the WADA Foundation Board, January 13, 2000, Lausanne, p. 5.

16. Pound, *Inside Dope*, 94–95.

17. Pound quoted in McCarthy, "Profile: Richard W. Pound, QC-Chairman of WADA," S20.

18. Minutes of the Inaugural Meeting of the WADA Foundation Board, January 13, 2000, Lausanne, p. 10.

19. Ibid., p. 13.

20. Fourteen decisions were made at the meeting. For historians, the most important of these was the agency's determination to make the minutes of its meetings publicly available on the WADA website. The decisions of the initial meeting are provided in the Minutes of the Inaugural Meeting of the WADA Foundation Board, January 13, 2000, Lausanne, p. 18.

21. See the IOC's description of the meeting in "World Anti-Doping Agency," *Olympic Review*, February–March 2000, 6.

22. Minutes of the Meeting of the WADA Foundation Board, March 22, 2000, Lausanne, p. 1.

23. Ibid., pp. 30, 34–35, 32, 24.

24. Syväsalmi quoted in Natasha Bita, "10,000 to Be Tested Ahead of Games," *The Australian*, March 23, 2000.

25. Minutes of the Meeting of the Executive Committee of the World Anti-Doping Agency, June 20, 2000, Lausanne, p. 4.

26. Ibid., p. 5.

27. Ibid., p. 7.

28. Ibid., p. 8. For the challenges confronting WADA as it attempted to create a universal anti-doping culture in the international sports system, see Girginov, "Creating a Corporate Anti-Doping Culture," 252–268.

29. Housman quoted in Jere Longman, "Olympics: New Olympic Doping Accusations Cast Shadow," *New York Times*, June 22, 2000.

30. Samaranch quoted in Amy Shipley, "IOC Moves to Close Drug-Testing Gap: Medical Panel Approves New Procedure for Detecting Endurance-Enhancing Drug Erythropoietin," *Washington Post*, August 2, 2000. The methods for detecting erythropoietin are outlined in Evanthia Diamanti-Kandarakis et al., "Erythropoietin Abuse and Erythropoietin Gene Doping: Detection Strategies in the Genomic Era," *Sports Medicine* 35, no. 10 (2005): 832–834.

31. Gosper quoted in Amy Shipley, "IOC Adds New Drug Test: Field for 2008 Games Narrowed to Five Cities," *Washington Post*, August 29, 2000.

32. Emphasis in original. Minutes of the Conference Call of the WADA Executive Committee, August 2, 2000, Lausanne, p. 7.

33. Ibid.

34. "The best Games ever," quoted from Harri Syväsalmi, "Preface," WADA Independent Observer Report, Olympic Games 2000, Sydney, http://www.wada-ama.org/en/. The subsequent quotations are from pages 1 and 2 of the report.

35. Ctvrtlik quoted from Minutes of the Informal Meeting of the WADA Foundation Board, September 15, 2000, Sydney, p. 4.

36. Rajiv Chandrasekaran, "Two Flunk IOC Drug Tests: Silver Medalist among Ejected," *Washington Post,* September 20, 2000.

37. The Bulgarian lifters who tested positive were women's gold medalist Izabela Dragneva, men's bronze medalist Sevdalin Minchev, and men's silver medalist Ivan Ivanov. See "Olympic Notebook: Entire Bulgarian Team Suspended," *Washington Post,* September 22, 2000. Ivanov's suspension is noted in Chandrasekaran, "Two Flunk IOC Drug Tests."

38. See Minutes of the Meeting of the WADA Foundation Board, November 14, 2000, Oslo, p. 7.

39. Exum also alleged that he was the subject of racial discrimination at the USOC. See Amy Shipley, "Drug Chief Resigns, Blasts USOC," *Washington Post,* June 15, 2000.

40. See "Former Drug Testing Chief Sues USOC," *Physician and Sportsmedicine* 28, no. 9 (September 2000): 15.

41. Quoted in Hoberman, *Testosterone Dreams,* 256–257. "Lacks a credible international and national reputation" from Exum complaint, p. 11, John Hoberman personal research archive, University of Texas at Austin. Hoberman served as an expert witness for Exum.

42. See Kim Clark and Robert Milliken, "Positive on Testing," *U.S. News and World Report,* August 14, 2000, 40.

43. See Catriona Dixon, "Drop in Testing Alleged," *Daily Telegraph* (Sydney), September 6, 2000.

44. McCaffrey and Pound quoted in Amy Shipley, "U.S. Won't Underwrite Anti-Doping Agency: America Already Gives Enough, McCaffrey Says," *Washington Post,* September 13, 2000.

45. Heiberg quoted in Jere Longman, "Sydney 2000: Drug Testing. U.S. Goes on Offensive over Tests for Drugs," *New York Times,* September 27, 2000.

46. Ljungqvist quoted in Longman, "Sydney 2000."

47. Ljungqvist quoted in "IAAF: U.S. Not Coming Clean," *Washington Post,* October 2, 2000.

48. Masback quoted in Amy Shipley, "U.S. Track Official Defends Handling of Drug Tests," *Washington Post,* September 29, 2000. The proposal that WADA assume control of USA Track and Field's anti-doping efforts is outlined in Amy Shipley, "Overseer of Track Drug Plan Sought," *Washington Post,* September 30, 2000; and Richard Sandomir, "Sydney 2000: Track Group Proposes Compromise on Testing," *New York Times,* September 29, 2000.

49. Shorter quoted in John Meyer, "U.S. Drug Issue Grows: Agencies Disagree over Testing Control," *Denver Post,* September 29, 2000.

50. Pound quoted in Shipley, "Overseer of Track Drug Plan Sought."

51. Minutes of the Meeting of the WADA Foundation Board, November 14, 2000, Oslo, pp. 23–24. A short description of the decision is also provided in "USA Track and Field Criticized," *Washington Post,* November 15, 2000.

52. Pound quoted in Duncan Mackay, "Athletics: Doping Chief Calls for US to Be Expelled," *Guardian* (London), February 5, 2002.

53. Mannelly and Blackmun quoted in Thomas Heath, "USOC Plans to Polish Its Image," *Washington Post,* December 2, 2000.

54. See "Decisions" and comments by Denis Coderre in Minutes of the Informal Meeting of the WADA Foundation Board, September 15, 2000, Sydney, p. 4.

55. Vanstone remarks in Minutes of Meeting of the WADA Executive Committee, November 13, 2000, Oslo, p. 1.

56. Ibid., pp. 4–5.

57. See "Genomics and Its Impact on Science and Society: The Human Genome Project and Beyond" (2003), http://www.ornl.gov/sci/techresources/Human_Genome/publicat/primer2001/index.shtml.

58. See Miah, *Genetically Modified Athletes.* The perceptions of WADA chair Dick Pound regarding gene doping are articulated in Pound, *Inside Dope,* 179–188.

59. Robert Parienté, "After the Olympic Congress, on for Another Hundred Years," *Olympic Review,* October 1994, 402.

60. Schamasch quoted in Jere Longman, "Pushing the Limits—A Special Report: Someday Soon, Athletic Edge May Be from Altered Genes," *New York Times,* May 11, 2001.

61. Ljungqvist quoted in Longman, "Pushing the Limits."

62. Minutes of the Meeting of the WADA Executive Committee, March 6, 2001, Lausanne, p. 2.

63. Greene quoted in Longman, "Pushing the Limits."

64. Pound quoted in Richard Sandomir, "Olympics: Athletes May Next Seek Genetic Enhancement," *New York Times,* March 21, 2002. Pound's recollections of the meeting are provided in Pound, *Inside Dope,* 181–183.

65. See Saugy et al., "Human Growth Hormone Doping in Sport," 135–139.

66. Beginning in 1924, the Summer and Winter Olympic Games were held during the same year; the new format began with the 1994 Lillehammer Games.

67. Four of the seven had already signed contracts with WADA. These were the International Ski Federation, the International Bobsleigh and Skeleton Federation, International Luge Federation, and International Biathlon Federation. See Minutes of Meeting of the WADA Foundation Board, November 14, 2000, Oslo, p. 7.

68. Ibid., p. 20.

69. Discussions regarding a permanent headquarters were first conducted at the inaugural meeting of the WADA Foundation Board: Minutes of the Inaugural Meeting of the WADA Foundation Board, January 13, 2000, Lausanne, pp. 22–23.

70. Minutes of the Meeting of the WADA Executive Committee, November 13, 2000, Oslo, p. 14.

71. Coderre quoted in James Christie, "Montreal Ideal for Drug Watchdog, Experts Say: World Anti-Doping Agency Has Chance to Break European Mould in HQ Selection," *Globe and Mail* (Toronto), August 21, 2001.

72. The six finalists for the WADA headquarters were Vienna, Austria; Bonn, Germany; Lille, France; Lausanne, Switzerland; Stockholm, Sweden; and Montreal, Canada. Reference to them is made in Minutes of the Meeting of the WADA Foundation Board, November 14, 2000, Oslo, p. 9. The final vote for Montreal is provided in

Minutes of the Meeting of the WADA Foundation Board, August 21, 2001, Tallinn, Estonia, p. 7.

73. Coles quoted in Jere Longman, "On the Olympics: Samaranch's Complex Legacy," *New York Times,* July 10, 2001. As its title suggests, this article also provides a succinct analysis of Samaranch's legacy. See also Harry Gordon, "Samaranch and History . . . An Inheritance Very Different from the One He Received," *Journal of Olympic History* 9, no. 3 (September 2001): 5–6.

74. Quoted in Jere Longman, "Olympics: 3 Who Head Field in Competition to Lead the Olympic Movement," *New York Times,* April 5, 2001.

75. Ibid.

76. Pescante quoted in Amy Shipley, "IOC Leaning toward Rogge: Belgian Has Broad Support," *Washington Post,* July 15, 2001. A post-election sketch of the new IOC president is provided in Miguel Tasso, "Jacques Rogge: In the Name of Sport and Ethics," *Olympic Review,* August–September 2001, 35–38.

77. Jacques Rogge, "Towards Greater Universality," *Olympic Review,* August–September, 2001, 3.

78. Rogge quoted in James Stevenson, "Pound Returns to Anti-Doping Agency: IOC President Jacques Rogge Also Asking His Former Rival to Come Back as Marketing Chief," *Gazette* (Montreal), August 4, 2001.

79. Pound quoted in Christopher Smith, "Pound Praises Rogge on Doping Position," *Salt Lake Tribune,* February 15, 2002.

CHAPTER 10

1. Both the information on government funds and Pound's quote are from Amy Shipley, "Like Athletes, Anti-Doping Agency Gears Up for Games," *Washington Post,* January 18, 2002.

2. Quoted in William Booth, "Officials Promise 'Cleanest' Games Ever," *Washington Post,* February 10, 2002.

3. See Shipley, "Like Athletes, Anti-Doping Agency Gears Up for Games."

4. See Richard Sandomir, "Olympics: Tests Have Been Started for Banned Substances," *New York Times,* January 18, 2002; Janet Rae Brooks, "Doping Rears Its Ugly Head at Winter Games," *Canadian Medical Association Journal* 166, no. 6 (March 2002): 794.

5. Mitt Romney, *Turnaround: Crisis, Leadership, and the Olympic Games* (Washington, DC: Regnery, 2004), 161.

6. See "New Doping Agent Made Olympic Debut," *Physician and Sportsmedicine* 30, no. 4 (April 2002), 4.

7. Jovanovic was suspended after testing positive for an anabolic steroid at the U.S Olympic trials in December 2001. See Skip Knowles, "Bobsledder Suspended for Games," *Salt Lake Tribune,* January 28, 2002. Hays quoted in John Henderson, "Sliders Livid at Federation's Claim That Information Not Specific," *Denver Post,* February 10, 2002. Supplement use by Canadian athletes at the 1996 Atlanta and 2000 Sydney Olympics is examined in Shih-Han Huang, Karin Johnson, and Andrew L. Pipe, "The Use of Dietary Supplements and Medications by Canadian Athletes at the

Atlanta and Sydney Olympic Games," *Clinical Journal of Sport Medicine* 16, no. 1 (January 2006): 27–33. In Atlanta, 69 percent of the those who participated in interviews reported using some form of dietary supplements; this figure had grown to 74 percent by the Sydney Games (see p. 27).

8. The arbitration ruling stated, "We were unimpressed by, and do not accept, [Jovanovic's] evidence as to the care he took about the taking of supplements. He did not approach the [U.S. federation], or any other body, for guidance. He did not take medical advice. He relied only upon his own research, which, as we have found, was considerably less thorough than he would have had us believe. He ignored warnings about the dangers of contamination given by a number of bodies. He expressed no contrition, and accepted no blame, but sought to blame the IOC, WADA and USADA but not himself for the predicament in which he now finds himself." Quoted in John Henderson and John Meyer, "February 8," *Denver Post,* February 8, 2002.

9. See Arbitration CAS ad hoc Division (OWG Salt Lake City 2002) 001, Prusis and the Latvian Olympic Committee (LOC)/International Olympic Committee (IOC), award of February 5, 2002, in Matthieu Reeb, ed., *Digest of CAS Awards/Court of Arbitration for Sport (CAS)*, vol. 3 (The Hague: Kluwer Law International, 2004), 573–580. The most pertinent text of the CAS opinion stated: "In the Panel's opinion, if autonomy is to have any real meaning that meaning must be that it is a matter for the relevant International Federation to decide how it deals with doping offences which come within its jurisdiction and what sanctions to impose. If it were otherwise, the International Federation's autonomy would be illusory." The IOC, on the other hand, "can withdraw a sport, a discipline or an event . . . , or it can even withdraw recognition from that International Federation" (p. 577).

10. Dale Brazao, "Pound Upset after Bobsledder Reinstated," *Toronto Star,* February 8, 2002.

11. Wood quoted in Brian Maffly, "Anti-Doping Agency Accused after Clearing Estonian Athlete," *Salt Lake Tribune,* February 3, 2002.

12. Ibid.

13. See Minutes of the Meeting of the WADA Executive Committee, December 2, 2001, Lausanne, pp. 7–11. See also Minutes of the Meeting of the WADA Foundation Board, December 3, 2001, Lausanne, pp. 6–9.

14. Verbruggen quoted in Mihir Bose, "Cycling Leader's Scathing Attack on Top Scientists for 'Blocking' Tests on EPO," *Daily Telegraph* (London), February 15, 2002.

15. Ljungqvist quoted in Bose, "Cycling Leader's Scathing Attack on Top Scientists for 'Blocking' Tests on EPO."

16. Pound quoted in Mihir Bose, "Unseemly Squabbles Threaten the Fight to Rid World Sport of Drug Menace," *Daily Telegraph* (London), March 22, 2002.

17. Carrard quoted in Bose, "Unseemly Squabbles Threaten the Fight to Rid World Sport of Drug Menace."

18. Pound quoted in Jack Todd, "Working to Clean Up Olympics: Rogge Makes Symbolic Peace with Pound at Anti-Dope Agency Opening," *Gazette* (Montreal), June 2, 2002.

19. World Anti-Doping Agency, "Independent Observers Report: 2002 Olympic Games, Salt Lake City," pp. 88–89.

20. Pound quoted in Todd, "Working to Clean Up Olympics: Rogge Makes Symbolic Peace with Pound at Anti-Dope Agency Opening."

21. Ibid.

22. Pound quoted in James Christie, "Tough Drug Code Faces Sport Bodies," *Globe and Mail* (Toronto), June 5, 2002.

23. See Minutes of the Meeting of the WADA Executive Committee, December 2, 2001, Lausanne, pp. 4–7. It should be noted that the idea of a WADA code had been in existence since the creation of the new agency. Both the Harmonisation Congress and Kuala Lumpur are discussed in World Anti-Doping Agency 2002 Annual Report, available on WADA website. The Meeting in Kuala Lumpur is discussed in S. Selvam, "Anti-Doping Gets Good Response," *New Straits Times* (Kuala Lumpur), April 24, 2002.

24. This process is discussed in World Anti-Doping Agency 2002 Annual Report, pp. 6–8, available on WADA website.

25. Copenhagen Declaration on Anti-Doping in Sport, adopted at World Conference on Doping in Sport in Copenhagen, March 2003, available on WADA website.

26. Copenhagen Declaration, sections 2, 3, and 4.

27. Pound, *Inside Dope*, 98–99.

28. Rogge quoted in "Rogge Puts Weight of IOC behind Anti-Doping Code," *Ottawa Citizen*, March 4, 2003.

29. Copenhagen Declaration, section 2.4. Athletic organizations were given an even more aggressive schedule. They were to adopt the World Anti-Doping Code by the 2004 Summer Olympics in Athens. See Susanna Loof, "IOC Approves Global Anti-Doping Code: Decision Means World's Countries Face Uniform Rules," *Ottawa Citizen*, July 5, 2003.

30. See Loof, "IOC Approves Global Anti-Doping Code: Decision Means World's Countries Face Uniform Rules."

31. Pound quoted in Steve Keating, "Anti-Doping Brawl Puts Cycling Body at Risk of Missing Athens Olympics," *Courier Mail* (Brisbane), October 8, 2003.

32. Pound quoted in "Drug Chief Rails at U.S. 'Disinterest'," *St. Petersburg Times*, November 19, 2003.

33. The text of the convention is provided at "International Convention against Doping in Sport," October 19, 2005, available through the WADA website.

34. Owen quoted in James Christie, "Anti-Doping Accord Okayed," *Globe and Mail* (Toronto), October 20, 2005.

35. Ibid.

36. See "Doping: Sweden Ratifies Convention," *Ottawa Citizen*, November 27, 2005.

37. The seven to ratify were Australia, New Zealand, Canada, Denmark, Sweden, Norway, and Monaco. This information, as well as Rogge's quote, from "IOC's Rogge Presses for Approval of Doping Code: Olympics," *Seattle Times*, February 8, 2006.

38. The date for the convention to become effective was rescheduled for February 1, 2007. See "Govt to Ratify Treaty against Sports Doping: Signing Seen as Key to 2016 Olympic Bid," *Daily Yomiuri* (Tokyo), December 24, 2006.

39. Pound quoted in McCarthy, "Profile," S20.

40. See Vicki Michaelis, "IOC Asks Italy for Criminal Doping Waiver during Games," *USA Today*, February 11, 2005.

41. Pescante quoted in Nathaniel Vinton, "I.O.C. Ends Opposition to Italy's Doping Laws," *New York Times*, October 29, 2005.

42. See Amy Shipley and Liz Clarke, "Italian Authorities Still Plan to Prosecute Substance Abuse Cases," *Washington Post*, February 7, 2006.

43. See U.S. Senate, Subcommittee on Consumer Affairs, Foreign Commerce and Tourism of the Committee on Commerce, Science, and Transportation, *Steroid Use in Professional Baseball and Anti-Doping Issues in Amateur Sports: Hearing before the Subcommittee on Consumer Affairs, Foreign Commerce and Tourism of the Committee on Commerce, Science, and Transportation,* 107th Congress, 2nd sess., June 18, 2002 (Washington, DC: U.S. Government Printing Office, 2005); U.S. House, *The Drug Free Sports Act of 2005: Hearings before the Subcommittee on Commerce, Trade, and Consumer Protection of the Committee on Energy and Commerce,* 109th Congress, 1st sess., May 18 and 19, 2005 (Washington, DC: U.S. Government Printing Office, 2005); U.S. Senate, Committee on Commerce, Science, and Transportation, *S. 529, To Authorize Appropriations for the U.S. Anti-Doping Agency,* 109th Congress, 1st sess., May 24, 2005 (Washington, DC: U.S. Government Printing Office, 2005); U.S. House, Hearing before the Committee on Government Reform, *Restoring Faith in America's Pastime: Evaluating Major League Baseball's Efforts to Eradicate Steroid Use,* 109th Congress, 1st, March 17, 2005 (Washington, DC), http://gpoaccess.gov/congress/index .html; U.S. Senate, *Hearing before the Committee on Commerce, Science, and Transportation on S. 1114, The Clean Sports Act of 2005, and S. 1334, The Professional Sports Integrity and Accountability Act,* 109th Congress, 1st sess., September 28, 2005 (Washington, DC: U.S. Government Printing Office, 2006).

44. President Bush remarked, "To help children make right choices, they need good examples. Athletics play such an important role in our society, but, unfortunately, some in professional sports are not setting much of an example. The use of performance-enhancing drugs like steroids in baseball, football, and other sports is dangerous, and it sends the wrong message—that there are shortcuts to accomplishment, and that performance is more important than character. So tonight I call on team owners, union representatives, coaches, and players to take the lead, to send the right signal, to get tough, and to get rid of steroids now." George W. Bush, Address before a Joint Session of the Congress on the State of the Union, January 20, 2004, http://presidency.ucsb.edu.ws/print.php?pid=29646.

45. See AP, "Jones (Six Months), Former Coach (63 Months) Sentenced to Prison," January 14, 2008, http://sports.espn.go.com/oly/trackandfield/news/story?id=3191954.

46. See "Swimming: China's Missing Children," *Sunday Times* (London), May 8, 2005; Nicole Jeffrey, "Stasi Agent Helps Chinese Team," *Australian,* February 16, 2005.

47. Clegg quoted in Jacob Leibenluft, "The Agony of Victory," Foreign Policy Web Exclusive, posted August 2007, http://www.foreignpolicy.com/story/cms.php ?story_id=3963.

48. For a pre-Games analysis along these lines, see Dali L. Yang and Alan Leung, "The Politics of Sports Anti-Doping in China: Crisis, Governance and International Compliance," *China: An International Journal* 6, no. 1 (March 2008): 121–148.

49. Elizabeth C. Economy and Adam Segal, "China's Olympic Nightmare," *Foreign Affairs* 87, no. 4 (August 2008): 47.

50. Tony Blair, "We Can Help China Embrace the Future," *Wall Street Journal,* August 26, 2008.

51. Liang Lijuan, *He Zhenliang and China's Olympic Dream* (Beijing: Foreign Languages Press, 2007), 474.

52. "Doping Controls at Beijing Games Most Extensive Ever," http://www
.ebeijing.gov.cn/BeijingInfo/NewsUpdate/OlympicNews/t978452.htm.

CONCLUSION

1. Minutes of the WADA Foundation Board, November 14, 2000, Oslo, p. 13.

2. Friedmann quoted in "Sports and Drugs: Are Stronger Anti-Doping Policies Needed?" *Congressional Quarterly Researcher* 14, no. 26 (July 23, 2004): 624.

3. World Anti-Doping Code, 2003, subsection 4.3.2 comment, available online through the WADA website.

4. A useful summary of these points is provided in John M. Hoberman, "The Doping of Everyday Life," *Boston Globe,* August 21, 2006. Clipping from John Hoberman personal papers, University of Texas at Austin. My thanks to Dr. Hoberman for providing me with a copy of this article.

5. The accepted ratio of testosterone to epitestosterone is described in C. Saudan et al., "Testosterone and Doping Control," *British Journal of Sports Medicine* 40, no. 1, Supplement I (July 2006): i23.

6. See, for instance, Donald A. Berry, "The Science of Doping," *Nature* (August 7, 2008): 692–693; and Werner Pitsch, "The 'Science of Doping' Revisited: Fallacies of the Current Anti-Doping Regime," *European Journal of Sports Science* 9, no. 2 (March 2009): 87–95.

7. Pound quoted in "Sports and Drugs," 624.

8. Glorioso quoted in Sandomir, "Olympics: Athletes May Next Seek Genetic Enhancement."

BIBLIOGRAPHY

The bibliography is divided into four sections: Archives, Internet Websites and Record Collections, Government Documents, and Other Sources (books, journal articles, court cases, newspaper articles, magazine articles, reports, and unpublished materials).

ARCHIVES

International Olympic Committee Library and Archives, Lausanne
    Medical Commission Records of the International Olympic Committee
    Minutes of the Meetings of the Executive Board of the International Olympic Committee
    Minutes of the Meetings of the General Sessions of the International Olympic Committee
United States Olympic Committee Library and Archives, Colorado Springs, Colorado
    F. Don Miller Papers
    Minutes of the Meetings of the Administrative Committee of the United States Olympic Committee
    Minutes of the Meetings of the Board of Directors of the United States Olympic Committee and Its Executive Committee
    Robert Kane Papers
University of Arkansas, Fayetteville, Arkansas
    [U.S. Department of State] Bureau of Educational and Cultural Affairs Historical Collection
University of Illinois at Urbana-Champaign Archives
    Avery Brundage Collection (microfilm edition)
University of Texas at Austin
    Dolph Briscoe Center for American History
        Steven Ungerleider Collection
    Professor John M. Hoberman Personal Research Archives
    H. J. Lutcher Stark Center for Physical Culture and Sport
        Todd-McLean Physical Culture Collection

Beijing International: The Official Website of the Beijing Government: http://www
.ebeijing.gov.cn/

Cold War International History Project at the Woodrow Wilson Center: http://www
.wilsoncenter.org/index.cfm?fuseaction=topics.home&topic_id=1409
Cold War Files

ESPN: www.espn.com

International Olympic Committee: http://www.olympic.org

United Nations Educational, Scientific and Cultural Organization Documents and
Publications: http://unesdoc.unesco.org/ulis/index.shtml

University of California at Santa Barbara American Presidency Project:
Bush, George W. Address before a Joint Session of the Congress on the State of the
Union, January 20, 2004: http://presidency.ucsb.edu.ws/print.php?pid=29646

World Anti-Doping Agency: http://www.wada-ama.org/en/
Minutes of the Meetings of the Executive Committee of the World Anti-Doping
Agency
Minutes of the Meetings of the Foundation Board of the World Anti-Doping
Agency
"The World Anti-Doping Code: The 2007 Prohibited List International Standard."

GOVERNMENT DOCUMENTS

Remarks by Congressman Henry A. Waxman, The International Olympic Committee Reform Act, *Congressional Record (Extension of Remarks)*. 106th Congress,
1st sess., vol. 145, April 12, 1999. Washington, DC: U.S. Government Printing Office: 1999.

Dubin, Charles. *Commission of Inquiry into the Use of Drugs and Banned Practices Intended to Increase Athletic Performance.* Ottawa: Canadian Government Publishing
Centre, 1990.

U.S. Congress. *Congressional Record (Extension of Remarks),* 106th Congress, 1st sess.,
vol. 145. Washington, DC: U.S. Government Printing Office, 1999.

U.S. Congress. House. Committee on Government Reform. *Restoring Faith in America's
Pastime: Evaluating Major League Baseball's Efforts to Eradicate Steroid Use: Hearing
before the Committee on Government Reform.* 109th Cong., 1st sess., March 17, 2005,
http://gpoaccess.gov/congress/index.html.

U.S. Congress. House. Committee on Energy and Commerce. *The Drug Free Sports
Act of 2005: Hearings before the Subcommittee on Commerce, Trade, and Consumer
Protection of the Committee on Energy and Commerce.* 109th Cong., 1st sess., May 18
and 19, 2005. Washington, DC: U.S. Government Printing Office, 2005.

U.S. Congress. Senate. Committee on Commerce, Science, and Transportation. *To
Authorize Appropriations for the U.S. Anti-Doping Agency: Hearing on S. 529.* 109th
Cong., 1st sess., May 24, 2005. Washington, DC: U.S. Government Printing Of-
fice, 2005.

———. *Hearing before the Committee on Commerce, Science, and Transportation on S. 1114, The Clean Sports Act of 2005, and S. 1334, The Professional Sports Integrity and Accountability Act.* 109th Cong., 1st sess., September 28, 2005. Washington, DC: U.S. Government Printing Office, 2006.

———. *Steroid Use in Professional Baseball and Anti-Doping Issues in Amateur Sports: Hearing before the Subcommittee on Consumer Affairs, Foreign Commerce and Tourism of the Committee on Commerce, Science, and Transportation.* 107th Cong., 2nd sess., June 18, 2002. Washington, DC: U.S. Government Printing Office, 2002.

U.S. Congress. Senate. Committee on the Judiciary. Subcommittee to Investigate Juvenile Delinquency of the Committee on the Judiciary. *Investigative Hearings on the Proper and Improper Use of Drugs by Athletes before the Subcommittee to Investigate Juvenile Delinquency of the Committee on the Judiciary Pursuant to S. Res. 56, Section 12.* 93rd Cong., 1st sess., June 18, July 12, 13, 1973. Washington, DC: U.S. Government Printing Office, 1973.

COURT CASES

Reynolds v. International Amateur Athletic Federation, 1992 U.S. App. LEXIS 14058 (U.S. 6th Cir., 1992).

Reynolds v. International Amateur Athletic Federation, 505 U.S. 1301 (U.S. Supreme Court, 1992).

Reynolds v. International Amateur Athletic Federation, 841 F. Supp. 1444 (S.D. Ohio, 1992).

Reynolds v. International Amateur Athletic Federation, 23 F.3d 1110 (U.S. 6th Cir., 1994).

OTHER SOURCES

"3 U.K. Athletes Sent Home in Doping Scandal." *Toronto Star,* July 30, 1992.

"11 Nations in Drug Test Accord." *New York Times,* December 14, 1989.

"86 Athletes Tested Positive." *New York Times,* January 11, 1985.

"After the Congress of the Association Internationale de Boxe Amateur." *Bulletin du Comité International Olympique,* September 1951, 16–17.

Allen, Karen. "Group's Anti-Drug Action 'Thrills' U.S. Swimming." *USA Today,* February 14, 1995.

Almond, Elliott, Julie Cart, and Randy Harvey. "The Olympic Dope Sheet Is Redefined." *Los Angeles Times,* November 13, 1983.

———. "Testing Has Not Stopped Use of Steroids in Athletics: Soviets Led the Way, but West Has Caught Up." *Los Angeles Times,* January 29, 1984.

Amdur, Neil. "Mounting Drug Use Afflicts World Sports." *New York Times,* November 20, 1978.

———. "Use of Caffeine Cited: Drugs Played an Olympic Role." *International Herald Tribune,* November 15, 1972.

———. "Wider Olympic Drug Abuse Is Seen." *New York Times,* January 30, 1977.

"The Anti-Doping Battle Is Making Good Progress." *Bulletin du Comité International Olympique,* May 1963, 43–44.

Asher, Mark, and Christine Brennan. "TAC Clears Reynolds of Steroid Use Charge: International Hearing His Next Hurdle." *Washington Post,* October 5, 1991.

"Athletes Want Drug Bans." *Courier-Mail* (Brisbane), September 26, 1991.

Auf der Maur, Nick. *The Billion-Dollar Game: Jean Drapeau and the 1976 Olympics.* Toronto: J. Lorimer, 1976.

Axthelm, Pete, and Frederick Kempe. "The East German Machine." *Newsweek,* July 14, 1980.

Barney, Robert Knight. "Mr. Samaranch Goes to Washington: Protecting IOC Stakes in the American Corporate World." In *Bridging Three Centuries: Intellectual Crossroads and the Modern Olympic Movement. Fifth International Symposium for Olympic Research,* edited by Kevin B. Wamsley, Scott G. Martyn, Gordon H. MacDonald, and Robert Knight Barney, 29–36. London, ON: International Centre for Olympic Studies, 2000.

Barney, Robert Knight, Stephen R. Wenn, and Scott G. Martyn. *Selling the Five Rings: The International Olympic Committee and the Rise of Olympic Commercialism.* Rev. ed. Salt Lake City: University of Utah Press, 2004.

Beamish, Rob, and Ian Ritchie. "From Fixed Capacities to Performance-Enhancement: The Paradigm Shift in the Science of 'Training' and the Use of Performance-Enhancing Substances." *Sport in History* 25, no. 3 (December 2005): 412–433.

———. "The Spectre of Steroids: Nazi Propaganda, Cold War Anxiety and Patriarchal Paternalism." *International Journal of the History of Sport* 22, no. 5 (September 2005): 777–795.

———. "Totalitarian Regimes and Cold War Sport: Steroid 'Übermenschen' and 'Ball-Bearing Females'." In *East Plays West: Sport and the Cold War,* edited by Stephen Wagg and David L. Andrews, 11–26. New York: Routledge, 2007.

Becker, Debbie, and Dick Patrick. "USOC Control of Testing Might Come after Atlanta." *USA Today,* October 6, 1995.

Beckett, A. H. "Misuse of Drugs in Sport." *British Journal of Sports Medicine* 12 (January 1979): 185–194.

Beckett, A. H., G. T. Tucker, and A. C. Moffat. "Routine Detection and Identification in Urine of Stimulants and Other Drugs, Some of Which May Be Used to Modify Performance in Sport." *Journal of Pharmacy and Pharmacology* 19, no. 5 (May 1967): 273–294.

Berendonk, Brigitte. *Doping Dokumente: Von der Forschung zum Betrug.* Berlin: Springer-Verlag, 1991.

Berkowitz, Steve. "Muddied Waters Cloud Swimmer's Case: Neither Foschi nor U.S. Swimming Happy with Penalty for Positive Drug Test." *Washington Post,* February 11, 1996.

Berlioux, Monique. "Femininity." *Lettre d'information/Newsletter/Carta información,* December 1967, 1–2.

Berry, Donald A. "The Science of Doping." *Nature* (August 7, 2008): 692–693.

Bita, Natasha. "10,000 to Be Tested Ahead of Games." *The Australian,* March 23, 2000.

Blackshaw, Ian S., Robert C. R. Siekmann, and Janwillem Soek, eds. *The Court of Arbitration for Sport, 1984–2004.* The Hague: TMC Asser Press, 2006.

Blackwell, Judith. "Discourses on Drug Use: The Social Construction of a Steroid Scandal." *Journal of Drug Issues* 21, no. 1 (Winter 1991): 147–164.

Blair, Tony. "We Can Help China Embrace the Future." *Wall Street Journal,* August 26, 2008.

Bondy, Filip. "Barcelona: Swimming. Too Good? Too Fast? Drug Rumors Stalk Chinese." *New York Times,* July 31, 1992.

Booker, Christopher. *The Games War: A Moscow Journal.* London: Faber and Faber, 1981.

Booth, William. "Officials Promise 'Cleanest' Games Ever." *Washington Post,* February 10, 2002.

Bose, Mihir. "Cycling Leader's Scathing Attack on Top Scientists for 'Blocking' Tests on EPO." *Daily Telegraph* (London), February 15, 2002.

———. "Unseemly Squabbles Threaten the Fight to Rid World Sport of Drug Menace." *Daily Telegraph* (London), March 22, 2002.

Brazao, Dale. "Pound Upset after Bobsledder Reinstated." *Toronto Star,* February 8, 2002.

Brennan, Christine. "Suspension on Foschi Is Lifted: U.S. Officials Reverse Ban on Swimmer." *Washington Post,* February 24, 1996.

———. "USOC Eyes Tougher Tests: Wants No-Notice Drug Tests in All Sports." *Washington Post,* September 9, 1995.

"British Find Method to Detect Steroids." *Los Angeles Times,* November 1, 1973.

Brooks, Janet Rae. "Doping Rears Its Ugly Head at Winter Games." *Canadian Medical Association Journal* 166, no. 6 (March 2002): 794.

Brooks, R. V., R. G. Firth, and N. A. Sumner. "Detection of Anabolic Steroids by Radioimmunoassay." *British Journal of Sports Medicine* 9, no. 2 (July 1975): 89–92.

Burstyn, Varda. *The Rites of Men: Manhood, Politics, and the Culture of Sport.* Toronto: University of Toronto Press, 1999.

Buti, Antonio, and Saul Fridman. *Drugs, Sport and the Law.* Mudgeeraba, Australia: Scribblers Publishing, 2001.

Cady, Steve. "Drug Testers Stiffen Olympic Procedures." *New York Times,* December 7, 1979.

"Cameron, Two Others Banned for Steroid Use." *Los Angeles Times,* July 31, 1976.

"Canadian Inquiry." *New York Times,* October 6, 1988.

Carlson, Lewis H., and John J. Fogarty. *Tales of Gold: An Oral History of the Summer Olympic Games Told by America's Gold Medal Winners.* Chicago: Contemporary Books, 1987.

Cha, Victor D. *Beyond the Final Score: The Politics of Sport in Asia.* New York: Columbia University Press, 2009.

Chandrasekaran, Rajiv. "Two Flunk IOC Drug Tests: Silver Medalist among Ejected." *Washington Post,* September 20, 2000.

Chappelet, Jean-Loup, and Brenda Kübler-Mabbott. *The International Olympic Committee and the Olympic System: The Governance of World Sport.* New York: Routledge, 2008.

"China to Investigate Doping." *New York Times,* December 1, 1994.

Christie, James. "Anti-Doping Accord Okayed." *Globe and Mail* (Toronto), October 20, 2005.

———. "'Do It Right' Anti-Drug Watchdog Warned: Future of Olympics on Line, Coderre Says." *Globe and Mail* (Toronto), January 13, 2000.

———. "Montreal Ideal for Drug Watchdog, Experts Say: World Anti-Doping

Agency Has Chance to Break European Mould in HQ Selection." *Globe and Mail* (Toronto), August 21, 2001.

———. "Tough Drug Code Faces Sport Bodies." *Globe and Mail* (Toronto), June 5, 2002.

"Christie Slams US Decision on Reynolds." *Herald Sun* (Melbourne), June 18, 1991.

Clark, Kim, and Robert Milliken. "Positive on Testing." *U.S. News and World Report*, August 14 2000.

"Commission Reports." *Olympic Review,* September–October, 1989.

"Commission Reports." *Olympic Review,* July 1991, 320–325.

Cole, C. L. "Testing for Sex or Drugs." *Journal of Sport and Social Issues* 24, no. 4 (November 2000): 331–333.

"Commission Reports." *Olympic Review,* September–October 1989, 441–446.

Coubertin, Pierre de. *Olympic Memoirs.* Lausanne: International Olympic Committee, 1997.

"Cycle Group Bans Use of Blood Doping." *New York Times,* January 19, 1985.

Da Costa, Norman. "Illegal Drug Use by Athletes Reported on Rise in Canada." *Toronto Star,* September 25, 1991.

"The Daily Dope Dialogue." *Track and Field News,* February 1985, 52.

Deford, Frank, Kostya Kennedy, and Richard Deitsch. "Just Say No." *Sports Illustrated,* December 16, 2002.

DeFrantz, Anita L. "Which Rules? International Sport and Doping in the 21st Century." *Houston Journal of International Law* 31, no. 1 (Fall 2008): 20–21.

De la Chapelle, Albert. "The Use and Misuse of Sex Chromatin Screening for 'Gender Identification' of Female Athletes." *Journal of the American Medical Association* 256, no. 14 (October 10, 1986): 1920–1923.

Denlinger, Ken. "Warfare on Drugs Increases." *Washington Post,* February 12, 1980.

Diamanti-Kandarakis, Evanthia, Panagiotis A. Konstantinopoulos, Joanna Papailiou, Stylianos A. Kandarakis, Anastasios Andreopoulos, and Gerasimos P. Sykiotis. "Erythropoietin Abuse and Erythropoietin Gene Doping: Detection Strategies in the Genomic Era." *Sports Medicine* 35, no. 10 (2005): 831–840.

Dimeo, Paul. "A Critical Assessment of John Hoberman's Histories of Drugs in Sport." *Sport in History* 27, no. 2 (June 2007): 318–342.

———. "Good Versus Evil? Drugs, Sport and the Cold War." In *East Plays West: Sport and the Cold War,* edited by Stephen Wagg and David L. Andrews. New York: Routledge, 2007.

———. *A History of Drug Use in Sport, 1876–1976: Beyond Good and Evil.* New York: Routledge, 2007.

———. *Making the American Team: Sport, Culture, and the Olympic Experience.* Urbana: University of Illinois Press, 1998.

Dimeo, Paul, and Thomas M. Hunt. "Saint or Sinner? A Reconsideration of the Career of Prince Alexandre de Merode, Chair of the International Olympic Committee's Medical Commission 1967–2002." Unpublished manuscript.

Dirix, Albert. "The Problems of Altitude and Doping in Mexico." *Bulletin du Comité International Olympique,* February 1967, 43–46.

Dixon, Catriona. "Drop in Testing Alleged." *Daily Telegraph* (Sydney), September 6, 2000.

Dodd, Mike. "USOC Ready to Approve No-Notice Drug Testing." *USA Today,* April 12, 1996.

Domer, Thomas Michael. "Sport in Cold War America, 1953–1963: The Diplomatic and Political Use of Sport in the Eisenhower and Kennedy Administrations." PhD diss., Marquette University, 1976.

Dong, Jinxia. *Women, Sport, and Society in Modern China: Holding Up More than Half the Sky.* Portland, OR: Frank Cass, 2003.

"Doping: Sweden Ratifies Convention." *Ottawa Citizen,* November 27, 2005.

"Doping, the International Olympic Committee and the Press." *Bulletin du Comité International Olympique,* November 1963, 59–60.

"Drug Chief Rails at U.S. 'Disinterest'." *St. Petersburg Times,* November 19, 2003.

"Drug Testing at Issue." *New York Times,* April 29, 1983.

"Drugs Used." *New York Times,* August 6, 1984.

Dyreson, Mark. *Crafting Patriotism for Global Dominance: America at the Olympics.* New York: Routledge, 2009.

———. "Globalizing the Nation-Making Process: Modern Sport in World History." *International Journal of the History of Sport* 20 (March 2003): 91–106.

———. *Making the American Team: Sport, Culture, and the Olympic Experience.* Champagne: University of Illinois Press, 1998.

"Early Deaths of Soviet Athletes Due to Steroids? Magazine Cites 59 Cases in Which Banned Drugs Proved Fatal at Young Age." *Los Angeles Times,* September 6, 1984.

Economy, Elizabeth C., and Adam Segal. "China's Olympic Nightmare." *Foreign Affairs* 87, no. 4 (August 2008), 47.

Edelman, Robert. *Serious Fun: A History of Spectator Sports in the U.S.S.R.* New York: Oxford University Press, 1993.

"Effect of Drugs to Aid Athletes Studied by U.S." *New York Times,* August 22, 1976.

"E. German Women's Success Stirs U.S. Anger." *New York Times,* August 1, 1976.

Elasas, Louis J., Arne Ljungqvist, Malcolm A. Ferguson-Smith, Joe Leigh Simpson, Myron Genel, Alison S. Carlson, Elizabeth Ferris, Albert de la Chapelle, and Anke A. Ehrhardt. "Gender Verification of Female Athletes." *Genetics in Medicine* 2, no. 4 (July–August 2000): 249–254.

Espy, Richard. "The Olympic Games: Mirror of the World." In *The Olympic Games in Transition,* edited by Jeffrey O. Segrave and Donald Chu, 407–418. Champaign, IL: Human Kinetics (1988).

"The Executive Board and the Summer IFs in Barcelona." *Olympic Review,* May 1991, 184–187.

"The Executive Board in Berlin." *Olympic Review,* October–November 1991, 488–490.

"Executive Board Meeting of December." *Olympic Review,* January 1988, 21–22.

Eyquem, Marie-Thérèse. "Women['s] Sports and the Olympic Games." *Bulletin du Comité International Olympique,* February 1961, 48–50.

Fair, John D. "Isometrics or Steroids? Exploring New Frontiers of Strength in the Early 1960s." *Journal of Sport History* 20, no. 1 (Spring 1993): 1–24.

Ferstle, Jim. "Evolution and Politics of Drug Testing." In *Anabolic Steroids in Sport and Exercise,* edited by Charles E. Yesalis, 363–413. 2nd ed. Champaign, IL: Human Kinetics, 2000.

"Find No Drug in Olympics Cycling Death." *Chicago Daily Tribune,* March 26, 1961.

Fischer, Marc. "Germany Has Everything—Except for Harmony." *Washington Post,* July 22, 1992.

———. "IOC Supports Idea of Berlin Games." *Washington Post,* January 23, 1990.

Fish, Mike. "Atlanta Games: 111 Days. Drug Test." *Atlanta Journal and Constitution,* March 30, 1996.

FitzGerald, Mary K. "The Court of Arbitration for Sport: Dealing with Doping and Due Process during the Olympics." *Sports Law Journal* 7 (Spring 2000): 213–242.

"Flying Laboratory Operational Soon." *Olympic Review,* January 1990, 6–8.

"Former Drug Testing Chief Sues USOC." *Physician and Sportsmedicine* 28, no. 9 (September 2000): 15.

"Foschi Cleared to Compete." *New York Times,* June 19, 1997.

Francis, Charlie, with Jeff Coplon. *Speed Trap: Inside the Biggest Scandal in Olympic History.* New York: St. Martin's Press, 1990.

Franke, Werner W., and Brigitte Berendonk. "Hormonal Doping and Androgenization of Athletes: A Secret Program of the German Democratic Republic Government." *Clinical Chemistry* 43, no. 7 (July 1997): 1262–1279.

Furthermore. *Washington Post,* February 13, 1995.

Furthermore. *Washington Post,* May 18, 1995.

Furthermore. *Washington Post,* September 1, 1997.

Gafner, Raymond, ed. *1894–1994, The International Olympic Committee. One Hundred Years—The Idea—The Presidents—The Achievements.* Vol. 2. Lausanne: International Olympic Committee, 1994.

Galluzzi, David. "The Doping Crisis in International Athletic Competition: Lessons from the Chinese Doping Scandal in Women's Swimming." *Seton Hall Journal of Sport Law* 10 (Winter 2000): 65–110.

Gaudard, Aurelie, Emmanuelle Varlet-Marie, Francoise Bressolle, and Michel Audran. "Drugs for Increasing Oxygen Transport and Their Potential Use in Doping: A Review." *Sports Medicine* 33, no. 3 (2003): 187–212.

Gems, Gerald. *The Athletic Crusade: Sport and American Cultural Imperialism.* Lincoln: University of Nebraska Press, 2006.

"Germanys Closer to Olympic Merger." *Washington Post,* August 13, 1990.

Getler, Michael. "E. Germans, Drugs: Hard Facts Missing." *Washington Post,* May 27, 1979.

Gilbert, Bil. "Drugs in Sport: High Time to Make Some Rules." *Sports Illustrated,* July 7, 1969.

———. "Drugs in Sport: Problems in a Turned On World." *Sports Illustrated,* June 23, 1969.

———. "Drugs in Sport: Something Extra on the Ball." *Sports Illustrated,* June 30, 1969.

Gilbert, Doug. *The Miracle Machine.* New York: Coward, McCann, & Geoghegan, 1980.

Girginov, Vassil. "Bulgarian Sport Policy, 1945–1989: A Strategic Relations Approach." *International Journal of the History of Sport* 26, no. 4 (March 2009), 515–538.

———. "Creating a Corporate Anti-Doping Culture: The Role of Bulgarian Sports Governing Bodies." *Sport in Society* 9, no. 2 (April 2006): 252–268.

Gold, Allan R. "Albertville '92: I.O.C. Looks at Use of Blood Tests." *New York Times,* February 7, 1992.

Goodhart, Philip, and Christopher Chataway. *War without Weapons*. London: W. H. Allen, 1968.

Goodwin, Michael. "U.S.O.C. to Seek More Tests for Drugs." *New York Times*, March 24, 1985.

Gordon, Harry. "Samaranch and History . . . An Inheritance Very Different from the One He Received." *Journal of Olympic History* 9, no. 3 (September 2001): 5–6.

Gore, Al. "Al Gore: Promoting Preventive Education." *Olympic Review*, February–March 1995, 42–45.

"Govt to Ratify Treaty against Sports Doping: Signing Seen as Key to 2016 Olympic Bid." *Daily Yomiuri* (Tokyo), December 24, 2006.

Guttmann, Allen. "The Cold War and the Olympics." *International Journal* 43 (Autumn 1988): 554–568.

———. *Games and Empires: Modern Sports and Cultural Imperialism*. New York: Columbia University Press, 1996.

———. *The Games Must Go On: Avery Brundage and the Olympic Movement*. New York: Columbia University Press, 1984.

———. *The Olympics: A History of the Modern Games*. 2nd ed. Urbana: University of Illinois Press, 2002.

———. "The Politics of the Olympic Movement." In *The Changing Politics of Sport*, edited by Lincoln Allison. Manchester: Manchester University Press, 1993.

Hage, Philip. "Caffeine, Testosterone Banned for Olympians." *Physician and Sportsmedicine* 10, no. 7 (July 1982): 15–17.

Hanstad, Dag Vidar, Andy Smith, and Ivan Waddington. "The Establishment of the World Anti-Doping Agency: A Study of the Management of Organizational Change and Unplanned Outcomes." *International Review for the Sociology of Sport* 43, no. 3 (September 2008): 227–249.

Harrison, Hope M. *Driving the Soviets Up the Wall: Soviet–East German Relations, 1953–1963*. Princeton, NJ: Princeton University Press, 2003.

Harvey, Randy. "IOC Official Questions Drug Testing in Track." *Los Angeles Times*, May 9, 1989.

Hayes, Mark, and Michael Hiestand. "Krabbe Case." *USA Today*, August 24, 1993, international edition.

Hazan, Barukh. *Olympic Sports and Propaganda Games: Moscow 1980*. New Brunswick, NJ: Transaction Books, 1982.

Heath, Thomas. "Drug Testing Performance Enhanced: High-Tech Equipment, Better Methods, but Will Abusers Slip Through?" *Washington Post*, April 23, 1996.

———. "USOC Plans to Polish Its Image." *Washington Post*, December 2, 2000.

Henderson, John. "Sliders Livid at Federation's Claim That Information Not Specific." *Denver Post*, February 10, 2002.

Henderson, John, and John Meyer. "February 8." *Denver Post*, February 8, 2002.

Herrmann, Peter. "Germany's 'Miracle Machine' Is Left in the Blocks." *New York Times*, November 4, 1990.

Hill, Christopher R. *Olympic Politics*. 2nd ed. Manchester, UK: Manchester University Press, 1996.

Hoberman, John M. "Amphetamine and the Four-Minute Mile." *Sport in History* 26, no. 2 (August 2006): 289–304.

———. "The Doping of Everyday Life." *Boston Globe*, August 21, 2006.

———. "History and Prevalence of Doping in the Marathon." *Sports Medicine* 37, no. 4/5 (2007): 366–388.

———. "How Drug Testing Fails: The Politics of Doping Control." In *Doping in Elite Sport: The Politics of Drugs in the Olympic Movement*, edited by Wayne Wilson and Edward Derse, 241–274. Champaign, IL: Human Kinetics, 2001.

———. *Mortal Engines: The Science of Performance and the Dehumanization of Sport.* New York: Free Press, 1992.

———. "Offering the Illusion of Reform on Drugs." *New York Times*, January 10, 1999.

———. *The Olympic Crisis: Sport, Politics, and the Moral Order.* New Rochelle, NY: A. D. Caratzas, 1986.

———. "The Reunification of German Sports Medicine, 1989–2002." *Quest* 45, no. 2 (May 1993): 277–285.

———. *Testosterone Dreams: Rejuvenation, Aphrodisia, Doping.* Berkeley: University of California Press, 2005.

———. "Toward a Theory of Olympic Internationalism." *Journal of Sport History* 22, no. 1 (Spring 1995): 1–37.

———. "The Transformation of East German Sport." *Journal of Sport History* 17, no. 1 (Spring 1990): 62–68.

Hoberman, John M., and Charles E. Yesalis. "The History of Synthetic Testosterone." *Scientific American*, February 1995, 76–82.

Houlihan, Barrie. "Anti-Doping Policy in Sport: The Politics of International Policy Coordination." *Public Administration* 77, no. 2 (Summer 1999): 311–334.

———. "Civil Rights, Doping Control and the World Anti-Doping Code." *Sport in Society* 7, no. 3 (Autumn 2004): 420–437.

———. *Dying to Win: Doping in Sport and the Development of Anti-Doping Policy.* 2nd ed. Strasbourg, France: Council of Europe Publishing, 2002.

———. "Harmonising Anti-Doping Policy: The Role of the World Anti-Doping Agency." In *Doping and Public Policy*, edited by John M. Hoberman and Verner Møller, 19–30. Odense: University Press of Southern Denmark, 2004.

———. "Mechanisms of International Influence on Domestic Elite Sport Policy." *International Journal of Sport Policy* 1 (March 2009): 51–69.

———. "Policy Harmonization: The Example of Global Antidoping Policy." *Journal of Sport Management* 13 (July 1999): 197–215.

———. *Sport and International Politics.* New York: Harvester Wheatsheaf, 1994.

Huang, Shih-Han, Karin Johnson, and Andrew L. Pipe. "The Use of Dietary Supplements and Medications by Canadian Athletes at the Atlanta and Sydney Olympic Games." *Clinical Journal of Sport Medicine* 16, no. 1 (January 2006): 27–33.

Hulme, Derick L. *The Political Olympics: Moscow, Afghanistan, and the 1980 U.S. Boycott.* New York: Praeger, 1990.

Hunt, Thomas M. "American Sport Policy and the Cultural Cold War: The Lyndon B. Johnson Presidential Years." *Journal of Sport History* 33 (Fall 2006): 273–297.

———. "Countering the Soviet Threat in the Olympic Medals Race: The Amateur Sports Act of 1978 and American Athletics Policy Reform." *International Journal of the History of Sport* 24 (June 2007): 804–826.

———. "Sport, Drugs, and the Cold War: The Conundrum of Olympic Doping Policy, 1970–1979." *Olympika: The International Journal of Olympic Studies* 16 (2007): 19–42.

Huntford, Roland. "Olympic Training: Inside Russia's Non-existent Camp." *Observer* (London), April 9, 1967.

"IAAF: U.S. Not Coming Clean." *Washington Post,* October 2, 2000.

"Important Medical Meetings This Autumn." *Olympic Review,* September 1991, 433.

"Inquiry to Last Several Weeks: Use of Roniacol Is Blamed for Death of Knud Jensen in Olympic Bike Race." *New York Times,* August 30, 1960.

"Inside the Olympic Medical Tent." *Physician and Sportsmedicine* 24, no. 6 (June 1996): 28.

"International Olympic Charter against Doping in Sport." *Olympic Review,* November 1988, 628–631.

"IOC Anti-Drug Agency on the Drawing Board." *Chicago Sun-Times,* August 20, 1998.

"I.O.C. Issues Doping Report." *New York Times,* August 4, 1980.

"IOC Says It Will Ignore 5 Positive Steroid Tests." *Atlanta Journal and Constitution,* November 28, 1996.

"IOC's Rogge Presses for Approval of Doping Code: Olympics." *Seattle Times,* February 8, 2006.

"IOC to Review Procedures to Stem Drug Test Suits." *Washington Post,* December 8, 1992.

Janofsky, Michael. "Barnes Claims Testing for Steroids Was Flawed." *New York Times,* November 7, 1990.

———. "Drug Plan Gains Approval." *New York Times,* November 25, 1988.

———. "Drug Use by Prominent Athletes Reported." *New York Times,* November 29, 1990.

———. "I.O.C. Criticizes Federation Steroids Rule." *New York Times,* September 8, 1989.

———. "Johnson Loses Gold to Lewis after Drug Test." *New York Times,* September 27, 1988.

———. "Olympics: Sophisticated Doping Begets More Testing." *New York Times,* July 19, 1992.

Janofsky, Michael, and Peter Alfano. "Drug Use by Athletes Runs Free Despite Tests." *New York Times,* November 17, 1988.

Jeffrey, Nicole. "Stasi Agent Helps Chinese Team." *Australian,* February 16, 2005.

Jennings, Andrew. *The New Lords of the Rings.* London: Simon & Schuster, 1996.

"Johnson Home in Disgrace: Canada Bans Him for Life. Can't Run for Country or Get Funds." *Los Angeles Times,* September 27, 1988.

Johnson, Molly Wilkinson. *Training Socialist Citizens: Sports and the State in East Germany.* Boston: Brill, 2008.

Johnson, William Oscar, and Anita Verschoth. "Testy Times in Germany." *Sports Illustrated,* March 9, 1992.

Judge, Edward H., and John W. Langdon, eds. *The Cold War: A History through Documents.* Upper Saddle River, NJ: Prentice Hall, 1999.

Kalinski, Michael I. "State-Sponsored Research on Creatine Supplements and Blood Doping in Elite Soviet Sport." *Perspectives on Biology and Medicine* 46, no. 3 (Summer 2003): 445–451.

Karpovich, Peter V. "Effect of Amphetamine Sulfate on Athletic Performance." *Journal of the American Medical Association* 170 (May 30, 1959): 558–561.

Kavanagh, Tricia. "The Doping Cases and the Need for the International Court of Arbitration for Sport (CAS)." *University of New South Wales Law Journal* 22 (Summer 1999): 721–745.

Keating, Steve. "Anti-Doping Brawl Puts Cycling Body at Risk of Missing Athens Olympics." *Courier-Mail* (Brisbane), October 8, 2003.

Keys, Barbara. *Globalizing Sport: National Rivalry and International Community in the 1930s.* Cambridge, MA: Harvard University Press, 2006.

———. "The Internationalization of Sport, 1890–1939." In *The Cultural Turn: Essays in the History of U.S. Foreign Relations,* edited by Frank A. Ninkovich and Liping Bu, 201–220. Chicago: Imprint Publications, 2001.

———. "Spreading Peace, Democracy, and Coca-Cola: Sport and American Cultural Expansion in the 1930s." *Diplomatic History* 28, no. 2 (April 2004): 165–196.

Kidd, Bruce, Robert Edelman, and Susan Brownell. "Comparative Analysis of Doping Scandals: Canada, Russia, and China." In *Doping in Elite Sport: The Politics of Drugs in the Olympic Movement,* edited by Wayne Wilson and Edward Derse, 153–188. Champaign, IL: Human Kinetics, 2001.

Killanin, Michael Morris. *My Olympic Years.* New York: William Morrow, 1983.

Kingdon, John W. *Agendas, Alternatives, and Public Policies.* 2nd ed. New York: Longman, 2003.

Kingsbury, Benedict, Nico Krisch, and Richard B. Stewart. "The Emergence of Global Administrative Law," *Law and Contemporary Problems* 68, no. 3/4 (Summer–Autumn 2005): 15–61.

Kirshenbaum, Jerry. "Steroids: The Growing Menace." *Sports Illustrated,* November 12, 1979.

Klein, Alan M. *Growing the Game: The Globalization of Major League Baseball,* reprint ed. New Haven, CT: Yale University Press, 2008.

———. *Sugarball: The American Game, the Dominican Dream.* New Haven, CT: Yale University Press, 1991.

Klein, Harvey G. "Blood Transfusions and Athletics: Games People Play." *New England Journal of Medicine* 312, no. 13 (March 1985): 854–856.

Knight, Athelia. "Arbitration Panel Rules for Foschi." *Washington Post,* April 9, 1996.

———. "USOC: Atlanta Too Soon for Stronger Drug Testing." *Washington Post,* October 6, 1995.

Knowles, Skip. "Bobsledder Suspended for Games." *Salt Lake Tribune,* January 28, 2002.

Kochakian, Charles D., and Charles E. Yesalis. "Anabolic-Androgenic Steroids: A Historical Perspective and Definition." In *Anabolic Steroids in Sport and Exercise,* edited by Charles E. Yesalis, 17–49. 2nd ed. Champaign, IL: Human Kinetics, 2000.

Kolata, Gina. "Asthma Medications: Not a Clear Advantage." *New York Times,* July 22, 2008.

Koller, Dionne. "From Medals to Morality: Sportive Nationalism and the Problem of Doping in Sports." *Marquette Sports Law Review* 19, no. 1 (Fall 2008): 91–124.

———. "How the United States Government Sacrifices Athletes' Constitutional Rights in Pursuit of National Prestige." *Brigham Young University Law Review* (Fall 2008): 1465–1544.

"L.A. Cyclist Says Other Nations Used Stimulants." *Los Angeles Times,* August 30, 1960.

LaFeber, Walter. *Michael Jordan and the New Global Capitalism,* expanded ed. New York: Norton, 2002.

"Lausanne Declaration." *Olympic Review,* February–March 1999, 17–18.

Legwold, G. "Blood Doping and the Letter of the Law." *Physician and Sportsmedicine* 13 (March 1985): 37–38.

"Letter from the Publisher." *Sports Illustrated,* June 23, 1969.

Levine, Benjamin D. "Should 'Artificial' High Altitude Environments Be Considered Doping?" *Scandinavian Journal of Medicine and Science in Sports* 16, no. 5 (October 2006): 297–301.

Lijuan, Liang. *He Zhenliang and China's Olympic Future.* Beijing: Foreign Languages Press, 2007.

Litsky, Frank. "Some U.S. Athletes Leave Games at Caracas amid Stiff Drug Tests." *New York Times,* August 24, 1983.

Longman, Jere. "Olympics: 3 Who Head Field in Competition to Lead the Olympic Movement." *New York Times,* April 5, 2001.

———. "Olympics: New Olympic Doping Accusations Cast Shadow." *New York Times,* June 22, 2000.

———. "On the Olympics: Samaranch's Complex Legacy." *New York Times,* July 10, 2001.

———. "Pushing the Limits—A Special Report: Someday Soon, Athletic Edge May Be from Altered Genes." *New York Times,* May 11, 2001.

———. "Sydney 2000: Drug Testing. U.S. Goes on Offensive over Tests for Drugs." *New York Times,* September 27, 2000.

———. "Track and Field: I.A.A.F. Reduces Doping Bans." *New York Times,* August 1, 1997.

Loof, Susanna. "IOC Approves Global Anti-Doping Code: Decision Means World's Countries Face Uniform Rules." *Ottawa Citizen,* July 5, 2003.

Lord, Craig. "China's Missing Children." *Sunday Times* (London), May 8, 2005.

Lorge, Barry. "IOC Gears Up to Detect Drugs, Ingenious Cheating in Moscow." *Washington Post,* June 1, 1979.

Lucas, John A. *Future of the Olympic Games.* Champaign, IL: Human Kinetics, 1992.

Ludwig, Jack Barry. *Five Ring Circus: The Montreal Olympics.* Toronto: Doubleday, 1976.

Lyberg, Wolf. *The IOC Sessions: 1956–1988, Volume 2—A Study Made by Wolf Lyberg, Former Secretary General of the NOC of Sweden.* N.p.: n.d.

Lyons, Richard D. "Expert Urges Ban on Blood Doping." *New York Times,* March 28, 1985.

MacAloon, John J. *This Great Symbol: Pierre de Coubertin and the Origins of the Modern Olympic Games.* Chicago: University of Chicago Press, 1981.

Mackay, Duncan. "Athletics: Doping Chief Calls for US to Be Expelled." *Guardian* (London), February 5, 2002.

Maennig, Wolfgang. "On the Economics of Doping and Corruption in International Sports." *Journal of Sports Economics* 3, no. 1 (February 2002): 61–89.

Maffly, Brian. "Anti-Doping Agency Accused after Clearing Estonian Athlete." *Salt Lake Tribune,* February 3, 2002.

Magdalinski, Tara. "Sports History and East German National Identity." *Peace Review* 11, no. 4 (December 1999): 539–545.

Mandelbaum, Michael. *The Meaning of Sports: Why Americans Watch Baseball, Football, and Basketball, and What They See When They Do.* New York: Public Affairs, 2004.

Mandell, Richard D. *A Munich Diary: The Olympics of 1972.* Chapel Hill: University of North Carolina Press, 1991.

Marvin, Carolyn. "Avery Brundage and American Participation in the 1936 Olympic Games." *Journal of American Studies* 16, no. 1 (April 1982): 81–105.

Matthews, George R. *America's First Olympics: The St. Louis Games of 1904.* Columbia: University of Missouri Press, 2005.

McCarthy, Michael. "Profile: Richard W. Pound, QC-Chairman of WADA." *Lancet* 366 (December 2005): S20.

McKenzie, Christopher. "The Use of Criminal Justice Mechanisms to Combat Doping in Sport." *Bond University Sports Law eJournal* (August 2007), http://epublications .bond.edu.au/slej/4/.

McLaren, Richard. "A New Order: Athletes' Rights and the Court of Arbitration at the Olympic Games." *Olympika: The International Journal of Olympic Studies* 7 (1998): 1–24.

"Medical Commission," *[IOC] Newsletter,* February 1968, 71–73.

Mehlman, Maxwell J., Elizabeth Banger, and Matthew M. Wright. "Doping in Sports and the Use of State Power." *St. Louis University Law Journal* 15 (2005/2006): 15–73.

Meyer, John. "U.S. Drug Issue Grows: Agencies Disagree over Testing Control." *Denver Post,* September 29, 2000.

Miah, Andy. *Genetically Modified Athletes: Biomedical Ethics, Gene Doping and Sport.* New York: Routledge, 2005.

Michaelis, Vicki. "IOC Asks Italy for Criminal Doping Waiver during Games." *USA Today,* February 11, 2005.

"Militarism, Sport, Europe: War without Weapons." Special Issue. *European Sport History Review* 5 (June 2003).

Miller, Andy, and M. A. J. McKenna. "Court Returns Medals, Changes Doping Scoreboard." *Atlanta Journal and Constitution,* August 5, 1996.

Miller, David. *Olympic Revolution: The Biography of Juan Antonio Samaranch.* Rev. ed. London: Pavilion, 1996.

Møller, Verner. *The Doping Devil,* trans. John M. Hoberman (Copenhagen: Books on Demand GmbH, 2008), http://www.scribd.com/doc/14022659/The-Doping-Devil.

———. "Knud Enemark Jensen's Death during the 1960 Rome Olympics: A Search for Truth?" *Sport in History* 25, no. 3 (December 2005): 452–471.

Molotsky, Irvin. "Justice Department Begins Investigation of Salt Lake Bid." *New York Times,* December 24, 1998.

Morgan, William J. "Cosmopolitanism, Olympism, and Nationalism: A Critical Interpretation of Coubertin's Ideal of International Sporting Life." *Olympika: The International Journal of Olympic Studies* 4 (1995): 79–91.

Mullegg, Gaston, and Henry Montandon. "The Danish Oarsm[e]n Who Took Part in the European Championships at Milan in 1950: Were They Drugged?" *Bulletin du Comité International Olympique,* July 1951, 25–26.

National Center on Addiction and Substance Abuse at Columbia University. *Winning at Any Cost: Doping in Olympic Sports.* New York, 2000.

"New Doping Agent Made Olympic Debut." *Physician and Sportsmedicine* 30, no. 4 (April 2002): 4.

Noble, Kate, Robert Kroon, and Tandy Nigel. "No Medals for the IOC." *Time South Pacific,* February 15, 1999.

Nynka, Andrew. "Ukrainian Scientist Details Secret Soviet Research Project on Steroids." *Ukrainian Weekly,* November 9, 2003.

"The Olympian Battle over hGH." *Sports Illustrated,* October 30, 1995, 17.

"Olympian Says Drug Use Heavy." *Chicago Tribune,* June 23, 1976.

"Olympic Athletes Cleared." *Washington Post,* February 25, 1980.

"Olympic Notebook: Entire Bulgarian Team Suspended." *Washington Post,* September 22, 2000.

"Olympics: Backing for Germans." *New York Times,* August 17, 1990.

"Olympic Sports Set to Unify Doping Rules, Penalties." *Washington Post,* June 22, 1993.

Orwell, George. "The Sporting Spirit." *Tribune* (London), December 14, 1945.

Oschütz, Frank. "Harmonization of Anti-Doping Code through Arbitration: The Case Law of the Court of Arbitration for Sport." *Marquette Sports Law Review* 12 (Spring 2002): 675–702.

Parienté, Robert. "After the Olympic Congress, on for Another Hundred Years." *Olympic Review,* October 1994, 401–403.

Pataki, Ladislav, and Lee Holden. *Winning Secrets: Confessions of a Soviet Bloc Sports Scientist.* N.p.: Training Management Systems, 1989.

Patrick, Dick. "IOC Drug Chief's Proposal Blasted." *USA Today,* February 1, 1999.

Patrick, Dick, and Gary Mihoces. "Krabbe Cleared to Run by German Federation." *USA Today,* March 31, 1993.

Payne, Michael. *Olympic Turnaround: How the Olympic Games Stepped Back from the Brink of Extinction to Become the World's Best Known Brand.* Westport, CT: Praeger, 2006.

Percy, E. C. "Chemical Warfare: Drugs in Sports." *Western Journal of Medicine* 133, no. 6 (December 1980): 478–484.

Pickeral, Robbi, and Rodney Page. "USOC asks FBI to Investigate Web Site." *St. Petersburg Times,* December 9, 1997.

Pitsch, Werner. "The 'Science of Doping' Revisited: Fallacies of the Current Anti-Doping Regime." *European Journal of Sports Science* 9, no. 2 (March 2009): 87–95.

Pius XII, H. H. "Let Us Condemn the Practice of Doping." *Bulletin du Comité International Olympique,* February 1956, 65.

Plymire, Darcy C. "Too Much, Too Fast, Too Soon: Chinese Women Runners, Accusations of Steroid Use, and the Politics of American Track and Field." *Sociology of Sport Journal* 16, no. 2 (June 1999): 155–173.

Pope, Steven W. "Rethinking Sport, Empire, and American Exceptionalism." *Sport History Review* 38 (2007): 110, 111.

Pound, Richard W. *Five Rings over Korea: The Secret Negotiations behind the 1988 Olympic Games in Seoul.* Boston: Little, Brown, 1994.

————. *Inside Dope: How Drugs Are the Biggest Threat to Sports, Why You Should Care, and What Can Be Done about Them*. Mississauga, ON: John Wiley & Sons Canada, 2006.

————. *Inside the Olympics: A Behind-the-Scenes Look at the Politics, the Scandals, and the Glory of the Games*. Etobicoke, ON: J. Wiley & Sons Canada, 2004.

————. "Reflections on Cheating in Sport." *Olympic Review*, August 1989, 390–391.

Pound, Richard W., and John M. Hoberman. "Olympic Roundtable." *Olympika: The International Journal of Olympic Studies* 10 (2001): 73–86.

Reeb, Matthieu. "The Court of Arbitration for Sport (CAS)." In *Digest of CAS Awards, 1986–1998*, edited by Matthieu Reeb, xxiii–xxxi. Berne: Staempfli SA, 1998.

————, ed. *Digest of CAS Awards/Court of Arbitration for Sport (CAS)*. Vol. 3. The Hague: Kluwer Law International, 2004.

Reich, Kenneth. *Making It Happen: Peter Ueberroth and the 1984 Olympics*. Santa Barbara, CA: Capra Press, 1986.

"Report from the Commissions." *Olympic Review*, November 1988, 615–621.

Rich, Vera. "Mortality of Soviet Athletes." *Nature* 311 (October 4, 1984): 402–403.

Rinehart, Robert E. "Cold War Expatriot Sport: Symbolic Resistance and International Response in Hungarian Water Polo at the Melbourne Olympics, 1956." In *East Plays West: Sport and the Cold War*, edited by Stephen Wagg and David L. Andrews, 45–63. New York: Routledge, 2007.

Riordan, Jim. "Playing to New Rules: Soviet Sport and Perestroika." *Soviet Studies* 42, no. 1 (January 1990): 133–145.

Robb, Sharon. "Burned: At the Munich Olympics of 1972, a Young Swimmer Named Rick DeMont Was Stripped of His Gold Medal Due to a Bureaucratic Error. Think That Sounds Like an Easy Fix? Not Even Close." *Splash: The Official Newsletter of United States Swimming*, April–May 2001, 8–9.

Rogge, Jacques. "Towards Greater Universality." *Olympic Review*, August–September 2001, 3.

"Rogge Puts Weight of IOC behind Anti-Doping Code." *Ottawa Citizen*, March 4, 2003.

Romney, Mitt. *Turnaround: Crisis, Leadership, and the Olympic Games*. Washington, DC: Regnery, 2004.

Rosen, Daniel M. *Dope: A History of Performance Enhancement in Sports from the Nineteenth Century to Today*. Westport, CT: Praeger, 2008.

Rosen, Karen. "Foschi Files Lawsuit in Steroid Case." *Atlanta Journal and Constitution*, February 6, 1996.

Rostaing, Bjarne, and Robert Sullivan. "Triumphs Tainted with Blood." *Sports Illustrated*, January 21, 1985.

Ryan, Allan J. "A Medical History of the Olympic Games." *Journal of the American Medical Association* 205 (September 9, 1968): 715–720.

————. "Use of Amphetamines in Athletics." *Journal of the American Medical Association* 170 (May 30, 1959): 562.

Salvulescu, J., B. Foddy, and M. Clayton. "Why We Should Allow Performance Enhancing Drugs in Sport." *British Journal of Sports Medicine* 38, no. 6 (December 2004): 666–670.

"Samaranch: Doping Is a Fact." *New York Times*, July 2, 2001.

Samaranch, Juan Antonio. "The Fight against Doping." *Olympic Review,* October–November 1998, 3.

———. "The IOC President's Speech at the Opening of the 97th Session." *Olympic Review,* July 1991, 308–312.

———. "Maintaining Our Impetus." *Olympic Review,* January 1990, 5.

Samaranch, Juan Antonio, and Robert Parienté. *The Samaranch Years: 1980–1994, Towards Olympic Unity.* Lausanne: International Olympic Committee, 1995.

Sandomir, Richard. "I.O.C.'s Drug Plan Criticized at Hearing." *New York Times,* October 21, 1999.

———. "Olympics: Athletes May Next Seek Genetic Enhancement." *New York Times,* March 21, 2002.

———. "Olympics: Tests Have Been Started for Banned Substances." *New York Times,* January 18, 2002.

———. "Sydney 2000: Track Group Proposes Compromise on Testing." *New York Times,* September 29, 2000.

Santos, J. Ferreira, and Mario de Carvalho Pini. "Doping." *Bulletin du Comité International Olympique,* February 1963, 56–57.

Saudan, C., N. Baume, N. Robinson, L. Avois, P. Mangin, and M. Saugy. "Testosterone and Doping Control." *British Journal of Sports Medicine* 40, no. 1, Supplement I (July 2006): i21–i24.

Saugy, M., N. Robinson, C. Saudan, N. Baume, L. Avois, and P. Mangin. "Human Growth Hormone Doping in Sport." *British Journal of Sports Medicine* 40, no. 1, Supplement I (July 2006): 135–139.

Scott, Jack. "Drugs in Sports." *Chicago Tribune,* October 24, 1971.

———. "It's Not How You Play the Game, but What Pill You Take." *New York Times,* October 17, 1971.

Selvam, S. "Anti-Doping Gets Good Response." *New Straits Times* (Kuala Lumpur), April 24, 2002.

Senn, Alfred Erich. *Power, Politics, and the Olympic Games.* Champaign, IL: Human Kinetics, 1999.

"The Seoul Games, Day 12 Notes: Johnson Advertisements Canceled." *Los Angeles Times,* September 28, 1988.

Shipley, Amy. "Drug Chief Resigns, Blasts USOC." *Washington Post,* June 15, 2000.

———. "IOC Adds New Drug Test: Field for 2008 Games Narrowed to Five Cities." *Washington Post,* August 29, 2000.

———. "IOC Leaning toward Rogge: Belgian Has Broad Support." *Washington Post,* July 15, 2001.

———. "IOC Moves to Close Drug-Testing Gap: Medical Panel Approves New Procedure for Detecting Endurance-Enhancing Drug Erythropoietin." *Washington Post,* August 2, 2000.

———. "Like Athletes, Anti-Doping Agency Gears Up for Games." *Washington Post,* January 18, 2002.

———. "Overseer of Track Drug Plan Sought." *Washington Post,* September 30, 2000.

———. "U.S. Track Official Defends Handling of Drug Tests." *Washington Post,* September 29, 2000.

———. "U.S. Won't Underwrite Anti-Doping Agency: America Already Gives Enough, McCaffrey Says." *Washington Post,* September 13, 2000.

Shipley, Amy, and Liz Clarke. "Italian Authorities Still Plan to Prosecute Substance Abuse Cases." *Washington Post,* February 7, 2006.

Simson, Vyv, and Andrew Jennings. *Dishonored Games: Corruption, Money and Greed at the Olympics.* New York: S.P.I. Books, 1992.

Smith, Christopher. "Pound Praises Rogge on Doping Position." *Salt Lake Tribune,* February 15, 2002.

Smith, Gene M., and Henry K. Beecher. "Amphetamine Sulfate and Athletic Performance." *Journal of the American Medical Association* 170 (May 30, 1959): 543–557.

"Some on U.S. Squad at Caracas Failed Drug Tests before Games." *New York Times,* August 27, 1983.

"Soviet Olympic Body in Study." *New York Times,* March 13, 1965.

"Speech by H. E. Mr Juan Antonio Samaranch, IOC President." *Olympic Review,* May–June 1990, 243.

"Speech by H. E. Juan Antonio Samaranch, President of the International Olympic Committee, Moscow, 21st November 1988." *Olympic Review,* December 1988, 669–671.

"Speech by H. E. Juan Antonio Samaranch, President of the IOC (93rd Session)." *Olympic Review,* March 1988, 82–84.

"Speech Given by Mr. Avery Brundage, President of the International Olympic Committee, June 23, 1964, at la Sorbonne in Paris." *Bulletin du Comité International Olympique,* August 1964, 48.

Spitzer, Giselher. "A Leninist Monster: Compulsory Doping and Public Policy in the G.D.R. and the Lessons for Today." In *Doping and Public Policy,* edited by John M. Hoberman and Verner Møller, 133–143. Odense: University Press of Southern Denmark, 2004.

"Sporting Scene." *National Review* 31, no. 41 (October 12, 1979): 1280.

"Sports and Drugs: Are Stronger Anti-Doping Policies Needed?" *Congressional Quarterly Researcher* 14, no. 26 (July 23, 2004): 613–636.

Starkman, Randy. "Athletes Call for Doping Crackdown on Chinese Runners." *Toronto Star,* August 23, 1993.

———. "Chinese Track Success Sparks Doping Questions." *Toronto Star,* August 17, 1993.

Stephenson, J. "Female Olympians' Sex Tests Outmoded." *Journal of the American Medical Association* 276, no. 3 (July 17, 1996): 177–178.

"Steroid Drug Tests to Be Held." *Chicago Tribune,* September 1, 1974.

"Steroids Are Out and Marks Are Down in Some Field Events." *Los Angeles Times,* September 9, 1974.

Stevenson, James. "Pound Returns to Anti-Doping Agency: IOC President Jacques Rogge Also Asking His Former Rival to Come Back as Marketing Chief." *Gazette* (Montreal), August 4, 2001.

Straubel, Michael S. "Doping Due Process: A Critique of the Doping Control Process in International Sport." *Dickinson Law Review* 106 (Winter 2002): 523–572.

"Swimmers' Drug Tests in Spotlight." *Washington Post,* July 28, 1992.

"Swimming: China's Missing Children." *Sunday Times* (London), May 8, 2005.

"Swimming: Foschi Is Banned by International Group." *New York Times,* June 25, 1996.

Tasso, Miguel. "Jacques Rogge: In the Name of Sport and Ethics." *Olympic Review,* August–September 2001, 35–38.

Tax, Jeremiah. "A Look at Both the Seemly and Seamy Sides of Avery Brundage." *Sports Illustrated,* January 16, 1984.

"Team Lifted after 2d Drug Test Is Failed." *New York Times,* September 24, 1988.

"Team Physiologist Claims Nearly All U.S. Weightlifters on Steroids." *Los Angeles Times,* July 16, 1972.

Terret, Thierry. "Sport in Eastern Europe during the Cold War." *International Journal of the History of Sport* 26, no. 4 (March 2009): 465–468.

Thomas, Damion. "'Is It Really Ever Just a Game?'" *Journal of Sport and Social Issues* 29, no. 3 (August 2005): 358–363.

Thomas, James E., and Laurence Chalip, eds. *Sport Governance in the Global Community.* Morgantown, WV: Fitness Information Technology, 1996.

Thomas, Robert McG., Jr. "U.S.O.C. Checking Use of Transfusions." *New York Times,* January 10, 1985.

"Those Exempted Have 'Passes'." *Los Angeles Times,* January 17, 1972.

Todd, Jack. "Working to Clean Up Olympics: Rogge Makes Symbolic Peace with Pound at Anti-Dope Agency Opening." *Gazette* (Montreal), June 2, 2002.

Todd, Jan, and Terry Todd. "Significant Events in the History of Drug Testing and the Olympic Movement: 1960–1999." In *Doping in Elite Sport: The Politics of Drugs in the Olympic Movement,* edited by Wayne Wilson and Edward Derse, 65–128. Champaign, IL: Human Kinetics, 2001.

Todd, Terry. "Anabolic Steroids: The Gremlins of Sport." *Journal of Sport History* 14, no. 1 (Spring 1987): 87–107.

———. "A History of the Use of Anabolic Steroids in Sport." In *Sport and Exercise Science: Essays in the History of Sports Medicine,* edited by Jack W. Berryman and Roberta J. Park. Urbana: University of Illinois Press, 1992.

———. "Sports RX: The Use of Human Growth Hormone Poses a Grave Dilemma for Sport." *Sports Illustrated,* October 15, 1984.

"Towards an Anti-Doping Charter." *Olympic Review,* August 1988, 350.

"Track and Field: African Official Seeks Help on Drug Detection." *New York Times,* September 7, 1993.

"Track and Field: I.A.A.F. Drops Appeal on Krabbe." *New York Times,* January 29, 1997.

"Trainer Says He Issued Cyclist Drug." *Chicago Daily Tribune,* August 29, 1960.

Tuschak, Beth. "British Want IOC Heads to Clarify Doping Rules." *USA Today,* November 6, 1992.

Ueberroth, Peter, with Richard Levin and Amy Quinn. *Made in America: His Own Story.* New York: Fawcett Crest, 1987.

Ungerleider, Steven. *Faust's Gold: Inside the East German Doping Machine.* New York: Thomas Dunne Books / St. Martin's Press, 2001.

"USA Track and Field Criticized." *Washington Post,* November 15, 2000.

"USOC Imposing Tougher Drug Tests." *St. Petersburg Times,* December 13, 1997.

"USOC Passes Stiff Antidrug Program." *USA Today,* April 15, 1996.

"U.S.O.C. to Begin Tests." *New York Times,* June 25, 1985.

"U.S. Olympic Group to Weight Drug Test Plan: 86 American Athletes Failed 1984 Screening." *Chronicle of Higher Education* (1985), 3.

"U.S. Track Olympians Pass Drug Tests." *New York Times,* July 18, 1984.

Vinocur, John. "East German Tale of Tyranny." *New York Times,* January 11, 1979.

Vinton, Nathaniel. "I.O.C. Ends Opposition to Italy's Doping Laws." *New York Times,* October 29, 2005.

Voy, Robert O., and Kirk D. Deeter. *Drugs, Sport, and Politics: The Inside Story about Drug Use in Sport and Its Political Cover-up, with a Prescription for Reform.* Champaign, IL: Leisure Press, 1991.

Waddington, Ivan. *Sport, Health, and Drugs: A Critical Sociological Perspective.* London: Taylor & Francis, 2000.

Wagner, Ulrik. "The World Anti-Doping Agency: Constructing a Hybrid Organisation in Permanent Stress (Dis)order?" *International Journal of Sport Policy* 1 (July 2009): 183–201.

Wakefield, Wanda Ellen. "Out in the Cold: Sliding Sports and the Amateur Sports Act of 1978." *International Journal of the History of Sport* 24 (June 2007): 776–795.

Ward, R. J., C. H. Shackleton, and A. M. Lawson. "Gas Chromatographic–Mass Spectrometric Methods for the Detection and Identification of Anabolic Steroid Drugs." *British Journal of Sports Medicine* 9, no. 2 (July 1975): 93–97.

"Weight Lifter Used Drug." *New York Times,* September 29, 1988.

Wenn, Stephen R. "Riding into the Sunset: Richard Pound, Dick Ebersol, and Long-Term Olympic Television Contracts." In *Bridging Three Centuries: Intellectual Crossroads and the Modern Olympic Movement. Fifth International Symposium for Olympic Research,* edited by Kevin B. Wamsley, Scott G. Martyn, Gordon H. MacDonald, and Robert Knight Barney, 37–50. London, ON: International Centre for Olympic Studies, September 2000.

Wenn, Stephen R., and Scott G. Martyn. "'Tough Love': Richard Pound, David D'Alessandro, and the Salt Lake City Olympics Bid Scandal." *Sport in History* 26, no. 1 (April 2006): 64–90.

Wiederkehr, Stefan. "'We Shall Never Know the Exact Number of Men Who Have Competed in the Olympics Posing as Women': Sport, Gender Verification and the Cold War." *International Journal of the History of Sport* 26, no. 4 (March 2009): 556–572.

Wilson, Harold E., Jr. "The Golden Opportunity: Romania's Political Manipulation of the 1984 Los Angeles Olympic Games." *Olympika: The International Journal of Olympic Studies* 3 (1994): 83–97.

Wilson, Wayne, and Edward Derse, eds. *Doping in Elite Sport: The Politics of Drugs in the Olympic Movement.* Champaign, IL: Human Kinetics, 2001.

Winner, Christopher P. "Sports Doping Crisis Faces a Crossroads." *USA Today,* September 28, 1998, international edition.

Witherspoon, Kevin B. *Before the Eyes of the World: Mexico and the 1968 Olympic Games.* DeKalb: Northern Illinois University Press, 2008.

Witt, Günter. "Mass Participation and Top Performance in One: Physical Culture and Sport in the German Democratic Republic." *Journal of Popular Culture* 18, no. 3 (Winter 1984): 159–174.

Wolff, María Tai. "Playing by the Rules? A Legal Analysis of the United States Olympic Committee–Soviet Olympic Committee Doping Control Agreement." *Stanford Journal of International Law* 25, no. 2 (Spring 1989): 611–646.

Wong, Glenn M. *Essentials of Sports Law.* 3rd ed. Westport, CT: Praeger, 2002.

"World Anti-Doping Agency," *Olympic Review,* February–March 2000, 5–6.

"The World Conference on Doping in Sport." *Olympic Review,* October–November 1998, 9.

Wrynn, Alison M. "'A Debt Was Paid Off in Tears': Science, IOC Politics and the Debate about High Altitude in the 1968 Mexico City Olympics." *International Journal of the History of Sport* 23, no. 7 (November 2006): 1152–1172.

———. "The Human Factor: Science, Medicine and the International Olympic Committee, 1900–70." *Sport in Society* 7, no. 2 (Summer 2004): 211–231.

Yang, Dali L., and Alan Leung. "The Politics of Sports Anti-Doping in China: Crisis, Governance and International Compliance." *China: An International Journal* 6, no. 1 (March 2008): 121–148.

Yesalis, Charles E., ed. *Anabolic Steroids in Sport and Exercise.* 2nd ed. Champaign, IL: Human Kinetics, 2000.

Yesalis, Charles, and Virginia S. Cowart. *The Steroids Game.* Champaign, IL: Human Kinetics, 1998.

Zeiler, Thomas W. *Ambassadors in Pinstripes: The Spalding World Baseball Tour and the Birth of the American Empire.* Lanham, MD: Rowman and Littlefield, 2006.

INDEX

Numbers in italics refer to photographs.

de Merode, Prince Alexandre (*continued*)
international anti-doping effort,
83–84, 85, 167n93; and doping cover-
ups, 75–76, 79–80, 164nn29,36; and
IOC medical commission, 23–24, 27,
28, 148n95, 156n8; and IOC public relations, 92; on leaking of test results,
58; on out-of-competition testing, 89,
94; on postcompetition sanctions and
punitive measures, 56, 107, 148n92;
and regulatory jurisdiction, 27, 28,
32–34, 36–37, 40, 67, 91, 106
DeMont, Rick, 39, 45–46, 47, 50
Denmark, 6, 7, 11, 43, 64. *See also* Jensen,
Knud
Dennis, Evie, 68
Dexedrine, 136–137
Diadora, 80
Dianabol, 9, 58
Dickson, Thomas, 77
dietary supplements, 179–180n7, 180n8
Diop, I. M., 157n37
Dirix, Albert, 146n68, 148n95
diuretics, 118
Donike, Manfred, 66, 67, 79, 163n17
Dooley, H. Kay, 21
doping: and allowable drugs and "soft
doping," 44, 45, 47–48, 62, 137,
154n44, 154n44; definition of, 3,
12, 15, 27, 145n45; education about,
23, 93–94, 126; encouraged by state
governments, 7, 25–26, 38, 39, 50
(*see also specific countries*); history of
(pre-1960), ix, 10, 143n21; as means
of qualifying for Olympics, 56–57;
Olympic policies and regulation
regarding (*see* International Olympic
Committee [IOC]); penalties for, 24,
27, 28, 43, 48, 57, 78, 89–90, 92–93,
97, 104–105, 114, 148n92; physical and
health effects of, 10, 24, 53–54, 79;
relationship of, to nationalism, patriotism, and the "spirit of sport," x, 3–4,
7, 39, 50–53, 59, 60, 78–79 (*see also*
Cold War; nationalism); responsibility of coaches and physicians in, 21,
65, 83, 103; scandals and cover-ups of,

3, 6, 45–47, 62, 67–69, 71, 75–76, 119,
169n22; substances used in, 5, 22, 36,
50, 76–77 (*see also* altitude training;
"blood doping"; gender cheating);
testing for (*see* testing). *See also specific
drugs/performance enhancers; and
specific Games*
Doping Dokumente (Berendonk), 92
Dragneva, Izabela, 177n37
Dreschler, Heike, 169n30
drugs, performance enhancing. *See*
doping
drugs, recreational, 21–22, 115
Dubin, Charles, 82–83
Dugal, Robert, 64, 157n37
Duncan, Sandy, 27–28
Dupre, Paul, 94
Dyreson, Mark, 139–140n3

Eastern Europe: doping in, 50, 94–95;
sport as means of political power in,
3, 84, 140–141n11. *See also* Cold War;
Soviet-bloc countries; *and specific
countries*
East Germany. *See* German Democratic
Republic (GDP)
Eklund, Bo, 10, 16
ephedrine, 24, 44, 45, 82
epitestosterone, 66
ergogenic aids. *See* doping
erythropoietin (EPO), 94, 116, 170n43;
new form of, 127; screens for, 121, 125,
127
Estonia, 126
ether, 44
European Amateur Athletic Federation,
55
European Athletics Championships, 32
European Council on Doping, 16
Ewald, Manfred, 73
Exum, Wade, 118, 120, 177n39

Fahey, John, 132
Falsetti, Herman, 76
Fantini, Sergio, 170n41

FBI, 104
Fédération Internationale de Basketball Amateur, 48
Fédération Internationale de Natation (FINA). *See* International Swimming Federation (FINA)
Fédération Internationale de Médecine du Sport (FIMS), 14, 23
First Travel Corporation, 72
Food and Drug Administration, 165n42
Foschi, Jessica, 104–105
France, 106
Francis, Charlie, 79, 80
Franke, Werner, 92
Fraysse, Mike, 69, 164–165n40
Freeh, Louis, 104
Freidman, Theodore, 136
Friedrich, Heike, 169n30

gender cheating, 29–32, 34, 35–36, 43–44, 149–150n26
genetic manipulation (genomics), x, 5, 111, 121–122, 136
German Democratic Republic (GDR): and Chinese doping, 100; and nationalist conception of sport, 50–52, 156n10; Olympic success of, 51, 53, 59–60; perception of athletes of, 58–59; state-sponsored doping program of, 4, 39, 50, 53–54, 63, 92–93, 95, 109, 160n14; test results and penalties for athletes of, 58–59, 95, 97, 161n32, 169n30; threat of, to Soviet Union, 51–53, 73–75
Germany (unified), 92; swimming federation of, 102; and tension between East and West sports organizations, 95, 170–171n49; and testing in South Africa, 95–97
Giegenbach, Bob, 57
Gilbert, Bill, 3, 37
Glasnost, 84
Glorioso, Joseph, 137
Gorbachev, Mikhail, 81, 84–85
Gore, Al, 103
Gosper, Kevan, 116

Gramov, Marat, 73–74
Grau, Sigrun, 95
Great Britain, 84
Greene, Maurice, 122
Gresko, Anatoly, 161n32
Grippaldi, Phil, 57
Grut, Wille, 46, 47
Gummel, Margitta, 53

Hains, General, 49–50
Hale, Ralph, 103
hallucinogens, 22
Hanley, Daniel, 57; and altitude training, 19; call of, for standardization of testing, 28, 41, 43; conflict of interest between roles of, 50; and gender testing, 31; on testing in 1980 Moscow Games, 63
Hase, Dagmar, 169n30
Hay, Eduardo, 24, 34, 35, 36, 67, 148n95, 165n44
Hays, Todd, 126
Heiberg, Gerhard, 119
Heidebrecht, Larry, 80–81
Henderson, Paul, 114, 115, 136
hermaphrodites, 43. *See also* testing: for gender
heroin, ix
Hess, Norman, 64s
He Zhenliang, 134
Hicks, Thomas, 10, 11
Hiltner, Michael, 6
Hinze, Kurt, 51
Hoberman, John, 164n29, 170–171n49
Hoffman, Bob, 7–8
Höppner, Manfred, 53
hormones, 28, 44. *See also* gender cheating; *and specific hormones*
Housman, Rob, 116
Howald, Hans, 163n17
Howman, David, 121
Human Genome Project, 121
human growth hormone (hGH), 73, 122, 136, 173n23
Humphrey, Hubert, 22
Hungary, 53, 82, 140–141n11

Hunter, C. J., 119
Hybl, Bill, 104

Independent Observers Program, 117
International Amateur Athletics Federation, 67, 119
International Amateur Swimming Federation, 30
International Association of Athletics Federations (IAAF), 30, 67–68, 79, 85, 90–91, 97, 105
International Biathlon Federation, 178n67
International Bobsleigh and Skeleton Federation, 126, 178n67
International Boxing Federation, 7
International Cycling Union, 17, 44, 48, 127, 130
International Luge Federation, 178n67
International Olympic Charter against Doping, 98
International Olympic Committee (IOC): anti-American sentiment in, 46; anti-doping code of, 106, 115, 128, 130 (*see also* World Anti-Doping Code); anti-doping programs and policies of, 3, 11, 17, 22–25, 40, 43, 49, 54, 62, 67, 77–78, 83–85, 88–89, 92–94, 95–96; and bribery, allegations of, 106, 112, 174n47; and Court of Arbitration for Sport (CAS), 89–90, 105, 106, 126, 180n9; and doping, passivity toward, 6–7, 9–10, 43, 69, 77, 92–93, 101; doping subcommittee of, 12–15, 24; and enforcement of anti-doping policy (*see* testing); financial concerns of, 40, 71–73, 76, 91, 92–93, 125–126; and jurisdiction (*see* regulatory jurisdiction); leadership of, ix, x, 5, 49, 71, 106, 123–124, 135 (*see also specific leaders*); list of prohibited substances by, 2, 22, 24, 28–29, 46–47, 50, 54, 67, 105, 106, 147n78, 157n38, 159–160n4; and medical commission (*see* International Olympic Committee medical commission); and national govern-

ments, 2–4, 34–35, 83–84, 97–98, 102, 105, 131–132, 141n17; and sports federations, 7, 15–17, 32–35, 39–41, 47, 78, 79, 83, 88, 90, 102, 105, 126 (*see also specific federations*). See also doping
International Olympic Committee *Bulletin*. See *Bulletin du Comité International Olympique*
International Olympic Committee medical commission, 166n72; conflicts of interest in, 50; and implementation of testing, 56–58; members of, 148n95; perception of, as overzealous, 73, 85; regulatory power of, 24–25, 27, 32–36, 39–41, 47, 67, 106, 117, 167n93; and Rick DeMont, 45–46, 47; and sports physicians, 50, 156n8; and World Anti-Doping Agency (WADA), 117. *See also* de Merode, Prince Alexandre
International Rowing Federation, 7
International Sailing Federation, 114
International Ski Federation, 127, 178n67
International Swimming Federation (FINA), 101, 105, 172n6
International Weightlifting Federation, 117
Italy, 84, 131–132
Ivanov, Ivan, 177n37

Jacomini, Enrico, 97
James, David, 50
Jennings, Andrew, 66, 161n27
Jensen, Knud, 6, 7, *8,* 10, 11, 26, 136
Johnson, Ben, *81;* effect of, on doping practice and policy, 62, 83, 89, 101, 109–110, 136; positive test for steroids of, 4, 79, 80–83, 148n92
Jones, Marion, 119, 132
Jones, William, 48
Jorgensen, Oluf, 6
Jovanovic, Pavle, 126, 179–180n7, 180n8

Kaczmarek, Zbigniew, 58
Kalinski, Michael, 65
Kammerer, Craig, 76, 164n36

Kapitan, Boleslaw, 57–58

Kelly, Jack, 68

Killanin, Lord Michael Morris, 30, 47, 49, 58, 135

Klein, Harvey, 77

Koch, Marita, 52

Korneev & Gouliev v. International Olympic Committee, 173n35

Krabbe, Katrin, 95–97, *96*, 171n55

Krickow, Dieter, 47

Krieg, Pierre, 14

Krumm, Philip, 57

Kuala Lumpur: and the International Intergovernmental Consultative Group against Doping in Sport, 129

Kyodo Oil Company, 80

La Cava, Giuseppe, 148n95

LaShutka, Greg, 90

Latvia, 126

Lausanne Declaration, 107

Lewis, Carl, 75, 80

Lin Li, 100

Livingston, Jason, 171n57

Ljungqvist, Arne, 119, 121, 127, 165n56

Lockwood, Dean, 57

Lucas, Charles, 10–11

Lyon, Dave, 80

Mannelly, Matthew, 120

Marder, Alois, 160n13

marijuana. *See* cannabis

Masback, Craig, 119

Mayer, Otto, 12, 14, 15, 16

McCaffrey, Barry, 107, 108, *108*, 114, 118

McPhee, Harry, 19

Michaels, Jeff, 161–162n41

Mikhaylova, Birginia, 165n56

Miller, F. Don, 63, 71, 77

Minchev, Sevdalin, 177n37

Misersky, Henrich, 51

modern pentathlon, 46–48

Moller, Silke, 170n48

Møller, Verner, 143n21

Moran, Mike, 118

Moses, Edwin, 80

Moyer, Norman, 116, 123

nandrolone, 119, 126

Nantel, Albert, 157n37

National Broadcasting Company, 175n11

National Collegiate Athletic Association, 19

National Collegiate Track Coaches Association, 143n16

National Institutes of Health, 77

nationalism, 38, 41, 140–141n11, 151nn2,3; effect of, on doping, 3–4, 7, 39, 50–53, 59, 60, 78–79

National Security Council, 1

Nebiolo, Primo, 68, 76

Netherlands, the, 48, 49, 54; and Harmonisation Congress, 129

Neufeld, Renate, 63

nicotinamide, 50

Nitkin, Semyon, 161n32

norandrosteron, 126

Norway, 84

Nurikian, Norair, 95

Oberholzer, Alberto, 6

Observer, The (London), 20

Olympic Council of Asia, 101, 172n9

Olympic Games, modern: broadcasting of, 111, 175n11; and changing of schedule, 122, 178n66; creation of, ix; doping in (*see* doping); financial considerations of, 71–73, 76, 88, 92–93, 111 (*see also* testing: cost of); motto of, ix; as site of national rivalry and power struggle, 2–3, 9 (*see also* Cold War; nationalism). *See also* International Olympic Committee (IOC); *and specific Games*

Olympic Health Services (Los Angeles), 72

Olympic Review, 88, 124

Olympic Sports Medicine Committee, 59

opiates, 24

Oral-Turinabol, 53

Orwell, George, 39
O'Shea, Pat, 45
Otto, Kristin, 169n30
Owen, Stephen, 130

Pan Pacific Swimming Association, 102
Parienté, Robert, 121
Pataki, Ladislav, 53
Patano, Patty, 72
Patera, Ken, 42–43
Paulen, Adrian, 55
Payne, Michael, 72
Pells, Leah, 101
People's Daily, 102
People's Republic of China (PRC), 87, 132; and 2008 Beijing Games, 132–134; and accusations of racism, 101, 172n9; post–Cold War doping in, 100–102, 133, 172n6
performance enhancement. *See* doping
Pescante, Mario, 123, 131–132
pharmaceuticals, 21–22. *See also specific drugs*
Philby, Kim, 161n32
Pittsburgh Human Gene Therapy Center, 137
Poland, 53
Pope Pius XII, x, 9
Popov, V. I., 161n32
Porritt, Arthur: on Avery Brundage, 12; and gender testing, 30–31; as head of IOC doping subcommittee, 14–15, 16, 17, 22–23, 145n43
Pound, Richard "Dick," *113,* 142n15; on Ben Johnson scandal, 62, 82, 83, 86, 105; on East German athletes, 51; on gene manipulation, 111, 122; on IOC doping policy, 87–88, 105, 106; on Jose Samaranch, 72, 124, 128; perception and personality of, 112–113, 123, 135–136; on regulatory jurisdiction, 108, 112, 126; on testing scandals, 68, 76; on testing at 2002 Salt Lake City Games, 125, 128; on United States, 120, 130; on value of sport, 112–113; and World Anti-Doping Agency

(WADA), 109, 112–113, 115, 116, 117, 118, 119–120, 123–124, 130; and World Anti-Doping code, 129, 130, 131
Powell, John, 79
probenecid, 79, 80
Prokop, Ludwig, 148n95
Prouty, David, 77, 78
Prusis, Sandis, 126
Puerto Rico, 48, 49

Radford, Peter, 93
Ramsay, Sam, 96–97
Ratjen, Herman, 29
Reagan, Ronald, 69
regulatory jurisdiction: fragmentation of, 2–4, 13, 17, 39, 44, 48, 60, 64, 89, 90, 91, 97, 104–106, 111–112, 117, 126–127, 135–136; IOC's denial of, 7, 15–16, 23–24, 25, 28, 32–35, 39–40; unification of, 4–5, 27, 35–36, 87–88, 91, 106–109, 122. *See also* International Olympic Committee (IOC); World Anti-Doping Agency (WADA)
Reynolds, Butch, 90–91, 169n24
Reynolds v. International Amateur Athletic Federation, 169nn24,28
Rhiel, Winston, 45
Roby, Douglas, 20
Rochat, Jean-Philippe, 105
Rogge, Jacques, 123–124, 128, 129–130, 131
Rogozhin, Victor, 62–63
Romania, 53, 117
Romney, Mitt, 125–126
Roniacol, 6
Rosen, Daniel M., 143n21
Royal College of Surgeons, 14

Saltin, Bengt, 127
Samaranch, Juan Antonio, *108;* and commercial and economic viability of Olympics, 76, 85, 88, 92–93, 111, 135; and consolidation of international anti-doping effort, 83–84; and doping cover-ups, 164n29; on IOC's list of

Lightning Source UK Ltd.
Milton Keynes UK
UKHW010625270122
397797UK00001B/21